An Atlas of the

Human Embryo and Fetus

A Photographic Review of Human Prenatal Development

THE ENCYCLOPEDIA OF VISUAL MEDICINE SERIES

An Atlas of the
Human Embryo and Fetus

A Photographic Review of Human Prenatal Development

Jan E. Jirásek, MD, DSc
Laboratory of Reproductive Embryology
Institute for the Care of Mother and Child
Prague, Czech Republic

Foreword by
Louis G. Keith, MD
Professor of Obstetrics and Gynecology
Northwestern University Medical School
Chicago, IL, USA

The Parthenon Publishing Group
International Publishers in Medicine, Science & Technology

NEW YORK   LONDON

Library of Congress Cataloging-in-Publication Data
  An atlas of the human embryo and fetus: a photographic review
of human prenatal development / Jan E. Jirásek.
       p. ; cm. – (The encyclopedia of visual medicine series)
  Includes bibliographic references and index.
  ISBN 1-85070-659-X
  1. Embryology, Human – Atlases. 2. Fetus – Atlases. 3. Fetus –
Growth – Atlases. I. Jirásek, Jan E. (Jan Evangelista) II. Series.
  [DNLM: 1. Embryo – Atlases. 2. Fetal Development – Atlases.
3. Fetus – Atlases. QS 617 A8815 2000]
  RG613 A855 2000
  612.6'4'00222--dc21
                      00-033639

British Library Cataloguing in Publication Data
  An atlas of the human embryo and fetus : a photographic review
  of human prenatal development. – (The encyclopedia of visual
  medicine series)
  1. Human embryo – Atlases 2. Fetus – Atlases
  I. Jirásek J. E.
  612.6'46
  ISBN 185070659X

Published in the USA by
The Parthenon Publishing Group Inc.
One Blue Hill Plaza
PO Box 1564, Pearl River
New York 10965, USA

Published in the UK and Europe by
The Parthenon Publishing Group Limited
Casterton Hall, Carnforth
Lancs., LA6 2LA, UK

Copyright © 2001 The Parthenon Publishing Group

Printed and bound by T.G. Hostench S.A., Spain

CONTENTS

FOREWORD

This book represents the amalgamation of genius and perseverance. Not since the Carnegie Collection has the medical world seen pictures such as are contained in this volume. Moreover, these illustrations are but a fraction of the images obtained by Professor Jirásek, MD, DSc, during his long and distinguished tenure as Professor of Embryology and Reproductive Medicine at the Institute for the Care of Mother and Child in Prague, The Czech Republic.

My first awareness of this collection occurred when Professor John J. Sciarra invited me to a special lecture at the Prentice Women's Hospital and Maternity Center in Chicago arranged to introduce Professor Jirásek to the senior faculty of Northwestern University. What was projected on videotape literally 'blew me away'. I was enormously impressed, not only by the lecture but also by the man who had formerly worked as Assistant Professor under Professor Sciarra when he (Dr Sciarra) was Chairman of the Department of Obstetrics and Gynecology at the University of Minnesota. The fact that both gentlemen had remained in contact all these years, even through the dreary days of the Communist regime in then Czechoslovakia, was the first chapter in the genesis of this volume.

The second began during a visit to Prague, when I stayed in a guestroom at the Institute for the Care of Mother and Child and met Professor Jirásek for a unique breakfast of sausages washed down with ice-cold Scotch prior to viewing his collection. Once dutifully fortified, we spent the entire morning viewing a multitude of specimens, slides, videos and photographs. It was soon apparent that this was a lesson in embryology nonpareil and never to be repeated.

The third and final chapter of the saga was to tell the whole story to Mr David Bloomer and to convince him that Professor Jirásek's material would represent a truly unique Atlas for the Parthenon Publishing Group. True to the Chinese adage that 'Fortune favours the prepared mind', David responded in the typical English manner that characterizes his business style (at least with me) – 'a wink, a nod and a shake of the hand'.

The author and publisher are to be congratulated. Each has completed his task admirably. The photos are culled from a vast collection and organized with great care. The reproduction quality is of the highest order. Many of the images are of structures never seen before. The readership for this volume should be wide and its shelf-life long. If I should venture a guess, this Atlas is destined to become a classic landmark in the field of embryology and an invaluable addition to our specialty.

Louis G. Keith, MD
Professor of Obstetrics and Gynecology
Northwestern University Medical School
Chicago, IL, USA

PREFACE

'Gnothi se auton.' *Socrates*

The aim of this book is to give everyone a pictorial insight into the history of his/her origin, which is very difficult to describe despite the fact that many textbooks of human embryology exist. Indeed, some descriptions can be quite inaccurate, and relatively few attempt to trace the pathways leading from genes under the influence of induction and interaction to the morphogenic development and finally to the phenotype of a human being.

The book is not necessarily laid out in a systematic fashion, and does not cover the development of all the organs. The digestive and endocrine systems, for example, are completely omitted. Photographs, optical micrographs and scanning electron micrographs are displayed throughout the ten chapters. The book begins with the pre-embryonic stage of development, during which fertilization triggers the mitotic potential of the oocyte. Cleavage of the oocyte creates two developmental systems: the nutritive, or trophoblastic, system develops from the externally located blastomeres while the inner cell mass derived from the internal blastomeres represents the primordium of the three primary germ layers, i.e. the ectoderm, the endoderm and the primary mesoderm. The formation of the germ layers is related to the differentiation of two apposed vesicles, the amniotic sac and the yolk sac, which are located within the trophoblast-covered chorionic vesicle (gestational sac). A flat, round area between the apposed amniotic sac and the yolk sac constitutes the embryonic disk. Development from the pre-embryo to the embryo is illustrated by the images of Chapters 1–3.

Chapter 4 follows the development of the embryonic mesoderm and the early organization of the embryo, based on the formation of the notochordal plate. During the third week, the notochordal plate induces differentiation of the neural groove. Then, interactions between the neuroectoderm, surface ectoderm and endoderm of the primitive digestive tube induce the formation of somites, which are involved in mechanisms closing the neural tube. At this stage, the beginning of the fourth week, the neuroectoderm and surface ectoderm become delineated. The neural-inducing role of the notochordal plate ends. The beating heart primordium appears between days 22 and 24 as the first intraembryonic functioning organ. At the end of the fourth week, the notochordal plate separates from the neural tube as well as from the endoderm of the early gut, and transforms into the notochord, delineated by a distinct capsule. The isolated notochord becomes an important axial organizing center for the spine, attracting two generations of sclerotomic mesenchyme: the first generation of cells released from somites provides material for the intervertebral disks, and the second released from isolated sclerotomes, after dermatomyotomes have differentiated, forms the cartilaginous vertebral primordia. Chapter 4 includes images related to the formation of somites, closure of the neural tube and separation of the notochord.

Chapter 5 deals with the external characteristics of human embryos, and illustrates the organization of the embryonic body into the head, the trunk and the extremities. The head is organized around the brain vesicles, and the mouth delineated by the jaws. The brain, derivative of the brain vesicles, is protected by the skull, the skeleton of the head. The trunk has cervical, thoracic, lumboabdominal and pelvic portions. Characteristic embryonic structures of the cervical portion of the body are the pharyngeal arches and pouches, related to the development of the thyroid gland, parathyroids and thymus. The skeleton of the neck consists of seven cervical vertebrae; the thoracic portion of the body is supported by 12 thoracic vertebrae, 12 ribs and the sternum, and contains the heart located within the pericardial cavity and the lungs within pleural cavities. The thoracic portion of the body is separated from the lumboabdominal portion by the muscular septum: the diaphragm. The lumboabdominal portion of the body contains the main derivatives of the endodermal digestive tube such as the stomach, the duodenum, the jejunoileum and most of the colon. In addition, other derivatives of the digestive tube are the liver and the pancreas. The digestive organs are located within the peritoneal cavity. Behind the peritoneal cavity, located retroperitoneally, are the adrenals and the kidneys. The lumboabdominal skeleton is contributed by five lumbar vertebrae. The lower portion of the peritoneal cavity is located in the pelvic portion of the body, supported by the pelvic girdle. The axial portion of the pelvis is contributed by five sacral vertebrae fused into the sacral bone, and five fused coccygeal vertebrae originally supporting the embryonic tail.

The pelvic organs include the terminal portion of the digestive tube and, preperitoneally, the urinary bladder and the urethra. In females, there are the ovaries, oviducts, uterus and vagina. In males, the prostate is located within the pelvis, while the testes are located externally within the scrotum under the penis.

During the embryonic stage, the most important changes of the external characteristics are related to the segmentation of the body, formation of the face and differentiation of the limbs. Images of the face and limbs are included in Chapters 7 and 8. Some highlights of fetal development using fetoscopy are presented in Chapter 6.

The embryonic heart is the principal organ establishing the integrity of the fetoplacental unit. The heart primordium, the heart tube, begins beating on about day 22–24 post-conception. The organogenesis of the heart is illustrated by the images of Chapter 9. Finally, Chapter 10 describes how the germ cells escape differentiation of the germ layers, and depicts the sex organs, especially the development of external genitalia.

The reader will be able to refer to the images included in the ten chapters of the book to answer such questions as: How does the human embryo appear at 14 days? At the end of the fourth week? At the end of the embryonic stage? Does the embryo appear human? What is the human face? Can the human being be defined? Even the experienced embryologist, by studying the images, will be able to compare historical ideas with photographic reality.

In spite of all our knowledge of genes, biochemistry and anatomy, I am fully aware that there is still much unknown about the pathways from genes to anatomical forms. Therefore, the following photographs illustrate just what I have seen, and I share with the reader images of wonderful creatures, images of cartilages, bones, heart and sex organs.

Every individual represents the mere expression of his/her genes, present in the DNA within every nucleus of the billions of his/her cells. What a miracle!

Jan E. Jirásek

ACKNOWLEDGEMENTS

I would like to express my gratitude to my friends who have helped me, during the past 40 years, to accumulate the embryos constituting my collection, which has served as material for this book, and to those who have provided outstanding technical assistance, or who gave me the opportunity to join them in the USA at the time of the divided world prior to 1989.

Those persons are my Czech co-workers, Dr J. Uher (deceased), B. Faltinová and Dr Z. Rychtr, and my American friends, Professors R. G. Gorlin, K. Prem, R. L. Shapiro and J. J. Sciarra.

I would like to thank many others for their support, especially at my Laboratory of Reproductive Embryology at the Institute for the Care of Mother and Child, Prague-Podolí, where most of the work was done.

I deeply appreciate working with Parthenon Publishing, especially with David G. T. Bloomer, Jean Wright and Dinah Alam whose efforts, artistic skills and editorial help made this book possible.

Jan E. Jirásek

GLOSSARY OF TERMS

AMH Anti-Müllerian hormone: substance inducing the regression of Müllerian ducts in male fetuses

Amnion Avascular fetal membrane formed by connective tissue, lined by cells of extraembryonic ectoderm (amniocytes)

Amniotic sac Ectodermal structure originating from inner cell mass of the blastocyst

Angiogenesis Growth of new vessels from pre-existing vessels

Apoptosis Programmed cell death

Artery A vessel transporting blood from the heart

Axial Located in the midline

Blastema Aggregate of cells: the interface between the blastema and surrounding cells is indistinct

Blastocyst Cavitated sphere consisting of external trophoectoderm and inner cell mass

Blastogenesis Formation of germ layers: ectoderm, endoderm and mesoderm

Capillary Tiny vessel: networks of capillaries are interposed between arteries and veins

Caudal In the direction of the tail

Cell System fulfilling physical conditions for life-related chemical reactions: a system of membranes and other molecular structures preventing free mixing of substances

Chondroskeleton Skeleton formed by cartilage

Chorion Embryonic envelope of the gestational sac consisting of chorionic plate and chorionic villi, formed from vascularized mesenchyme and trophoblast

Chromosome Single molecule of DNA linked with histones and proteins: visible in cells at mitosis. Each chromosome consists of a short arm and a long arm with an interposed centromere

Conception Fertilization of the oocyte

Conceptus All derivatives of the fertilized oocyte until birth

Diffusion Movement of molecules or ions in a fluid according to a physical gradient from areas of high to low concentration

Diploid Containing two chromosomal sets: one paternal and one maternal. A diploid human cell contains 46 chromosomes

Delivery Expulsion, or extraction, of a viable fetus

Dorsal In the direction of the spine

DNA Deoxyribonucleic acid: the coding molecule of genes; the memory molecule of life. The DNA molecule represents a long chain of nucleotides (containing deoxyribose) arranged into a double-stranded helix. Each chromosome contains one very long molecule of DNA

Ectoderm External, neural and protective, germ layer

Endocytosis Transport of substances into a cell across a cytoplasmic membrane

Endoderm Internal, digestive, germ layer

Epididymis Male organ apposed to the testis containing tubules transporting sperm

Epithelium Tissue consisting of closely packed cells: epithelia cover surfaces, glandular ducts, alveoli and tubules, or form trabeculae

Exocytosis Elimination of a substance from a cell across a cytoplasmic membrane

Fetal membranes Extraplacental amnion and chorion with apposed decidua

Frontal Perpendicular to sagittal and transverse, parallel to forehead

Gastrulation Formation of germ layers; term usually used instead of blastogenesis. In a strict sense, gastrulation means formation of gastrula, formation of endoderm

Germ layers Ectoderm (external), endoderm (internal) and mesoderm (intermediate): first tissues of the embryo

Gestation Time interval from the first day of the last menstrual period preceding conception until the expulsion of the conceptus by abortion or delivery: the normal length of human gestation until a full-term delivery is 280 days

Glycogen Intracellular polysaccharide consisting of glucose molecules

Haploid Containing only one set of chromosomes: mature germ cells are haploid, each chromosome representing a combination of paternal and maternal genes. The human haploid number of chromosomes is 23

hCG Human chorionic gonadotropin: hormonal glycoprotein of embryonic origin, produced by trophoblast

Life Phenomenon based on alternating selective and non-selective transcription of DNA. Selective transcription is coupled with coded RNA-related proteosynthesis. Non-selective DNA transcription means cellular division

Meconium Content of the fetal gut

Meiosis Two special divisions of terminally differentiated germ cells: at meiosis I, two diploid cells with a haploid number of chromosomes are formed; at meiosis II, each diploid cell from meiosis I divides into two haploid cells. Each chromosome of the haploid set exhibits a unique combination of paternal and maternal genes

Mesenchyme Loose embryonic connective tissue

Mesentery Attachment of the gut

Mesoderm Germ layer located between the ectoderm and the endoderm: gives rise to somites, nephric mesoderm, somatopleure and splanchnopleure

Mitosis Indirect division of cells. During mitosis, the doubled chromosomes of the paternal and maternal chromosomal set separate and constitute two diploid nuclei, which exhibit exactly the same DNA structure as the nucleus from which they originated. Subsequently, the cytoplasmic compartment between the newly formed nuclei splits by constriction of the cytoplasmic membrane. The phases of mitosis are: prophase, metaphase, anaphase and telophase

Morula Cleaved oocyte: aggregate of blastomeres surrounded by zona pellucida of the oocyte

Neuroepithelium   Early developmental stage of neural tissue: consists of cells preceding differentiation into neuroblasts, spongioblasts and ependyma

Organogenesis   Formation of the organs

Oocyte   Spherical female germ cell entering, or undergoing, meiosis

Placenta   Fetal organ performing all fetomaternal and maternofetal exchange. Connected with the fetus by the umbilical cord: represents a selective filter between maternal and fetal blood and has many additional endocrine and metabolic functions. The placenta is delivered and discarded after delivery of the fetus

Placode   Round or oval area containing specialized cells, located within the surface epithelium

Pronucleus   Nuclear-membrane-delineated compartment of the fertilized oocyte: two pronuclei are present after the second meiotic division of the oocyte has been completed. The male pronucleus contains the paternal chromosomal set; the female pronucleus contains the maternal chromosomal set

Proteosynthesis   Formation of proteins by the linking of molecules of amino acids

Raphe   Line of fusion

Rathke's pouch   Primordium of adenohypophysis: the anterior wall of Rathke's pouch is the area of primary fusion of neuroectoderm and surface ectoderm, close anteriorly to the prechordal plate of the trilaminar embryonic disk

Reticulum   Three-dimensional network of interconnecting stellate cells

Rostral   In the direction of the beak (nose)

RNA   Ribonucleic acid: effective molecule of proteosynthesis. The RNA molecule consists of nucleotides containing ribose. RNA molecules are single-stranded and are transcribed ('printed') on DNA

Sagittal   Arrowlike: in the anteroposterior direction perpendicular to the transverse and frontal planes

SEM   Scanning electron micrograph

Somite   Segment: mesodermal vesicle located lateral to the medullary tube

Spermatozoon   Mature, terminally differentiated, specialized haploid male cell produced by the testis

SRY   Male-determining region of Y chromosome, which triggers a chain of other genes related to the development of the testes

Stomodeum   Oral pit, early oral cavity

Testosterone   Male steroid sex hormone with anabolic properties, produced by testicular interstitial cells

Transverse   In the direction perpendicular to the frontal and sagittal planes

Trisomy   Presence of three, instead of two, chromosomes in a diploid chromosomal set

Trophoectoderm, trophoblast   Layer derived from external blastomeres of the cleaved oocyte: lining of the surface of chorionic, or placental, villi; the most important component of the placenta

Vasculogenesis   Formation of vascular networks from mesenchyme in situ

Vein   Vessel collecting blood from the capillaries and transporting it back to the heart

Ventral   In the direction of the abdomen

Yolk sac   Endodermal structure originating from the inner cell mass of the blastocyst

Zona pellucida   Spherical envelope of the oocyte, 15 μ in thickness, approximately 150 μ in diameter. It consists of glycoproteins

Zygote   Fertilized oocyte at the stage of first mitosis, after pronuclei have disappeared

SECTION ONE

A review of the human embryo and fetus

Introduction: the gestational period

Gestation begins with the first day of bleeding of the last menstrual period preceding fertilization. The average gestation extends over 280 days, 40 weeks or ten lunar months. Fertilization usually occurs on about day 14 of the menstrual cycle; therefore, the true anatomical age of the embryo or fetus is 14 days less than the gestational age. The average duration of prenatal development is 266 days. The average gestation is usually divided into several stages. The pregestation stage includes the days of the last menstruation and the days preceding fertilization. The pre-embyonic stage comprises fertilization, repeated divisions (cleavage) of the oocyte and formation of the hollow sphere known as the blastocyst. During this stage, the pre-embryo is transported from the ovary through the oviduct (Fallopian tube) into the uterus. On the 7th day after fertilization, the pre-embryo, or blastocyst, implants into the mucous membrane of the uterus. Implantation is regarded as the proper beginning of the embryonic stage. The blastocyst consists of two layers: an external layer of cells or trophectoderm (trophoblast) and an inner cell mass (embryoblast). After implantation, the inner cell mass of the blastocyst differentiates into two layers of embryonic cells, known as the external and internal germ layers (ectoderm and endoderm).

Formation of the three germ layers, between days 7 and 20, is known as blastogenesis, or gastrulation. This is followed by embryonic organogenesis, which takes place during developmental weeks 4–8. Segmentation of the embryonic body (formation of somites) is regarded as the beginning of organogenesis, while fusion of the rims of the eyelids is regarded as the end of embryonal organogenesis and ends the embryonal period. Developmental weeks 9–20, or gestational weeks 11–22, constitute the early stage. During this period, the fetus is considered to be unviable, and would not survive outside the uterus. At the end of gestational week 24, the average total body weight of the fetus is about 500 g. If such a fetus is delivered, there is a chance of its survival, and the survival rate increases with increasing total body weight. The normal full-term newborn is delivered at the end of the 40th gestational week. The average total body weight of a full-term newborn is about 3400 g; boys are heavier than girls.

The first 7 days of extrauterine life after delivery are known as the neonatal period, during which the newborn adapts from intrauterine to extrauterine conditions. Most importantly, oxygen provided previously to the fetus via the placenta is replaced postnatally by oxygen from the atmosphere via the lungs: the newborn begins to breathe.

CHAPTER 1

The pre-embryo: the journey from the ovary to the uterus

The phenomenon of life has existed on Earth for approximately 3.5 billion years. Therefore, although the genome of a new embryo is unique, the make-up of the embryo is not new. A human being originates from two living cells: the oocyte (female germ cell) and the spermatozoon (male germ cell), transmitting the torch of life to the next generation. The oocyte is a large cell, approximately 120μ in diameter, which develops a thick surrounding membrane, known as the zona pellucida. The diameter of the oocyte together with the zona is almost 0.2 mm (Figures 1.1 and 1.2). The spermatozoon is a small, very specialized male cell. The head of the spermatozoon, about 5μ in length with a diameter of about 3–4μ, contains the nucleus bearing the genetic information encoded within the DNA of the chromosomes. The spermatozoon moves, using the flagellum or tail, and the total length of the spermatozoon including the tail is about 60μ.

After release into the vagina, ejaculated spermatozoa swim up through the uterus and oviducts. Fertilization occurs at the abdominal end of the oviduct: a single spermatozoon penetrates the zona and is incorporated into the oocyte. Then, within the cytoplasm of the oocyte, the male and female pronuclei appear. The male pronucleus contains the paternal chromosomes and the female pronucleus contains the maternal chromosomes. Each chromosomal set in the pronuclei contains a unique combination of grandparental genes. Subsequently, the original, single set of chromosomes in each pronucleus doubles. The male and female pronuclei never fuse. As the oocyte divides, the chromosomes of the pronuclei, one set of maternal and one set of paternal origin, are transported into the nuclei of the first two cells, known as blastomeres. In tissue culture, during *in vitro* fertilization, the two first

blastomeres are present approximately 30–36 h after exposure of the oocyte to spermatozoa. Blastomeres contain the unique genome of a new individual. After fertilization, the oocyte divides (cleaves) repeatedly mitotically into blastomeres. The blastomeres become smaller and smaller, enclosed within the space limited by the zona of the original oocyte. The blastomeres, surrounded by the zona, represent the developmental stage known as the morula. At the stage of 16–20 blastomeres, those externally located join by intercellular junctions. Fluid accumulates within the centrally located cavity, and the morula becomes the blastocyst (Figure 1.3). The early blastocyst is a fluid-filled sphere. The originally external blastomeres develop into the trophoblast, while the group of internal blastomeres adheres locally to the internal surface of the trophoblast as the inner cell mass (embryoblast).

The morula is present on days 3 and 4, the blastocyst on days 5 and 6. Cleavage of the oocyte and formation of the blastocyst occur as the conceptus is transported through the oviduct (Figure 1.4) into the uterus. During this time, the large oocyte (the largest cell in the body) transforms into cells of normal somatic size.

As the blastocyst enters the uterus, and as its size enlarges, the zona of the original oocyte ruptures and is rejected. The blastocyst hatches, and, early in the 2nd week of development (days 7–8), implantation begins. The non-implanted conceptus, i.e. the fertilized oocyte, morula and free blastocyst, is designated the pre-embryo.

Much is known about pre-embryonic development as the result of *in vitro* fertilization (IVF) procedures. *In vitro* fertilization is a method used for the treatment of infertility, based on hormonal ovarian stimulation to produce oocytes. The oocytes are aspirated by an ultrasound-guided needle, placed into a tissue culture, inseminated, fertilized and further developed in tissue cultures. Pre-embryos exhibiting several blastomeres, or early blastocysts, are transferred into the uterus. Alternatively, in cases of male infertility, fertilization can be achieved under *in vitro* conditions by intracytoplasmic injection of a single spermatozoon using micro-manipulation.

CHAPTER 2

Implantation and the placenta

During day 7 post-fertilization, the trophoblast of the blastocyst adheres to the lining of the uterus, penetrating into the surface layer of the uterine mucous membrane and transforming into the trophoblastic shell. At the same time, the trophoblast begins to synthesize a specific hormone, human chorionic gonadotropin (hCG), which enters the maternal blood and is eliminated into the urine. This hormone is used as the basis for most pregnancy tests. On the trophoblastic shell, three zones can be distinguished: the inner, the middle and the peripheral. As the embryonic connective tissue (mesenchyme) develops, the trophoblastic shell, supported by mesenchyme, transforms into the chorion (Figure 2.1). The inner portion of the trophoblastic shell develops into the chorionic plate. As the mesenchyme of the chorionic plate grows into the middle zone of the trophoblastic shell, chorionic villi with mesenchymal stroma are formed (Figure 2.2). Between the villi is the intervillous space, which later contains maternal blood. The peripheral portion of the trophoblastic shell develops into the anchoring portions of the chorionic villi and into the peripheral trophoblast, which integrates with the decidual cells of the endometrium (uterine mucous membrane). The trophoblastic shell is present during the 2nd week of development. Transformation of the trophoblastic shell into the chorion, characterized by the presence of branching villi, takes place during the 3rd and most of the 4th week (Figures 2.3–2.7).

Until the end of the 4th week, the cells of the embryo are nourished by diffusion. Maternal blood penetrates into the intervillous space of the trophoblastic shell on about day 14, and, from days 15–16, maternal blood circulates within the intervillous space. The uterochorionic (later uteroplacental) circulation begins and, from now on, the trophoblast of chorionic villi is nourished from the maternal blood.

The embryonic heart begins beating on about day 22–23, accepting blood corpuscles from the yolk sac and pushing blood into the circulation. The embryonic blood begins circulating at the end of the 4th week of development. As a consequence of this embryochorionic circulation, the chorion differentiates into two portions: the villi of the frondous (villous) chorion are oriented against the uterine wall and are supplied by the embryonic, and later fetal, blood. They grow and branch, and form the villous portion of the chorion; the villi oriented towards the uterine cavity do not receive any fetal blood, and consequently degenerate into smooth avillous chorion. The size of the frondous chorion, the fetal portion of the future placenta, depends at this stage on the embryochorionic circulation, i.e. the efficiency of the fetal heart. Embryonic and later fetal blood is transported to the chorionic, and later to the placental, villi by two umbilical arteries (Figure 2.8). Blood returns from the chorion to the embryo and later to the fetus through a single umbilical vein. The two umbilical arteries and the single umbilical vein are located within the umbilical cord, which connects the abdomen of the embryo with the villous chorion, or placenta.

The start of the embryochorionic circulation changes the source of nourishment to all intra-embryonic tissues, including the chorionic mesenchyme. The survival and further development of the embryo become dependent on the circulation of embryonic/fetal blood. Establishment of the embryochorionic circulation represents the functional basis of the concept of the fetoplacental unit. If the embryochorionic circulation does not develop, or fails, the conceptus is aborted. The embryo cannot survive without the chorion (placenta), and the chorion will not survive without the embryo. Avascular degenerated chorionic villi constitute the hydatidiform mole (Figure 2.9).

The embryo develops within the amniotic sac, which is filled with amniotic fluid. As the embryo grows, the amnion expands. The space present temporarily between the chorionic plate and the amnion is the extraembryonic celom. The fusion of the amniotic mesenchyme with the mesenchyme of the chorion occurs between 10 and 12 gestational weeks. The extraembryonic space between the chorion and the amniotic sac disappears.

The placenta is diskoid, oval or round, with a diameter of approximately 20 cm, is 2–3 cm in thickness and weighs about 500 g at full term. The placenta, as well as the membranes, has a fetal and a maternal portion. The fetal portion of the placenta is derived from the villous chorion fused with the placental portion of the amnion. The maternal portion consists of the decidualized uterine mucous membrane and the intervillous space filled with maternal blood. The maternal surface of the placenta is lobular, each lobe consisting of two or three cotyledons. Each cotyledon represents a system of placental villi supplied by a terminal chorionic artery.

The fetal membranes are derived from the avillous chorion fused with the extraplacental amnion. The maternal surface of the membranes is covered by decidualized uterine mucosa. At parturition, the uterine mucosa splits. The placenta and membranes, together with the decidua (maternal in origin), are expelled from the uterus following delivery of the newborn. After delivery, only the basal layer of the uterine mucosa remains on the surface of the uterine cavity. The surface defect within the uterus heals during the following 6 weeks.

The placenta is a selective exchange barrier, mediating all maternofetal and fetomaternal transfers. The oxygen-rich maternal blood containing nutritive substances circulates within the intervillous space among the placental villi. The villi are covered by a continuous layer of trophoblast. Fetal vessels containing circulating fetal blood, which is oxygen-depleted and carries waste products of fetal metabolism, are located within the stroma of the villi. The maternal blood and fetal blood never mix, and are always separated by at least two layers of cells of fetal origin: the trophoblast and the lining of the fetal capillaries, the endothelium. Maternofetal and fetomaternal transfers are realized by various mechanisms. One of these is simple diffusion according to physical principles, which can be facilitated by 'channels' and transport proteins, and modified by water or lipid solubility. Other transport mechanisms include 'active' resorption, which requires energy; such transport takes place against physical gradients. Some substances, such as immunoglobulin G, including anti-Rh antibodies, which are related to immunity, cross the placental barrier by means of specific protein receptors. Mechanisms of exchange related to the transport of soluble big molecules across the trophoblast are known as endocytosis and exocytosis. In addition to its function in the exchange of water, oxygen, carbon dioxide, nutritive substances and metabolic waste, the placenta (trophoblast) is also a very potent endocrine organ. The most important hormones secreted by the placenta are hCG, human placental lactogen (hPL) and steroid hormones, such as estriol, estradiol and progesterone.

The most important enzymes of placental origin are placental alkaline phosphatase, diamine oxidase and cystine aminopeptidase.

The delivered placenta represents 500 g of living human cells which are usually discarded. The placenta may be a valuable source of human diploid cells, including blood stem cells.

CHAPTER 3

The embryo: blastogenesis, differentiation of the inner cell mass and formation of germ layers

The trophoblastic cells of the blastocyst and the inner cell mass represent two cell lines with different, independent developmental programs. While the trophoblastic blastomeres differentiate into the trophoblastic shell, or the future placenta, the blastomeres constituting the inner cell mass transform into three types of cells: ectodermal cells, endodermal cells and cells of the primary mesoderm (Figures 3.1–3.3). Interactions between ectodermal and endodermal cells of the inner cell mass result in the formation of two adjacent vesicles: the amniotic sac (formed by ectodermal cells) and the primary yolk sac (contributed by the endodermal cells) (Figure 3.2). The inner space of the blastocyst, between the trophoblastic shell and amniotic sac, and the yolk sac contain loose reticulum of primary mesoderm (Figure 3.3). A flat, round area bounded by the amniotic sac and yolk sac constitutes the embryonic disk, the 'anlage' or primordium of the embryo (Figures 3.4 and 3.5). The ectodermal cells of the embryonic disk are cylindrical and pseudostratified. At the end of the 2nd week, the endodermal cells of the disk already exhibit a marked 'craniocaudal gradient'. The cells at the head end of the embryo are cylindrical or cuboid, while the cells at the caudal (tail) end of the embryo are flat. Also at this stage, there is already a group of several large, round germ cells attached to the caudal ectodermal cells of the embryonic disk. These germ cells are stem cells for all the future spermatozoa in the testes, or the oocytes within the ovaries, and will be the only cells to be involved in the transmission of life to the next generation.

During the 3rd week, the chorion grows more rapidly than the amniotic sac and yolk sac (including the bilaminar embryonic disk). A fluid-filled space, the extraembryonic celom, appears within the primary mesoderm (mesenchyme) between the chorion and adjacent amniotic sac and yolk sac. At this stage, the conceptus consists of three vesicles: the chorionic vesicle or gestational sac containing the much smaller amniotic sac and yolk sac. The primary mesoderm condenses on the inner surface of the chorion and on the outer surfaces of the amniotic sac and yolk sac. A connecting stalk, a strand of mesenchyme between the caudal portion of the ceiling of the amniotic sac and the adjacent rim of the embryonic disk, attaches both embryonic vesicles to the chorion (Figure 3.6). Approximately on day 15, the organization of the embryonic disk is characterized by the appearance of midline (axial) structures. These are the primitive node (Hensen's node) and the primitive streak (Figures 3.7 and 3.8).

The primitive node appears within the ectoderm as a small agglomeration of cells, approximately in the middle of the bilaminar, round embryonic disk. This cellular aggregate provides a contact between the ectodermal and endodermal cells of the disk, and extends in a linear fashion to its caudal rim. This line of contact between the ectoderm and the endoderm, facilitated by adhesion molecules, is characteristic for the formation of the primitive streak. As a result of both the mitotic activity of the cells and the shift of cells from the ectoderm into the space between the ectoderm and the endoderm of the embryonic disk by way of the primitive

Specimens from this period of embryonic development are very rare. Unique micrographs are presented illustrating the disintegration of the primary yolk sac and closing of the secondary yolk sac. The black and white photographs of unsectioned human bilaminar and trilaminar embryos are the first of their kind.

streak, the primitive streak develops into the primitive groove (Figure 3.9). Attached to the caudal end of the primitive groove is a small area of closely apposed ectoderm and endoderm, without intervening 'mesoderm': the cloacal membrane. Trilaminar embryonic disks are pear-shaped (Figure 3.10).

The mesoderm is the third (middle) germ layer. Formation of the embryonic mesoderm results from the transformation of ectodermal epithelial cells into a multilayered sheath of cells located between the ectoderm and the endoderm. The cells of the embryonic mesoderm fill the space between the ectoderm and the endoderm of the germ disk, apart from the midline area anterior to the primitive node. A narrow cellular cord of polarized cells forming a tubule grows in a rostral fashion from the primitive node. This is known as the notochordal (chordomesodermal) process, or notochordal canal, which extends to the prechordal plate at the rim of the germ disk. Endodermal cells of the prechordal plate adhere closely to the overlying ectoderm and do not allow the process to extend any further. The notochordal process becomes incorporated into the ceiling of the yolk sac as the notochordal plate, by apoptosis of attached endodermal cells of the yolk sac and ventral cells of the notochordal canal. The notochordal canal changes into the notochordal plate.

The cells originally located within the ectoderm of the bilaminar germ disk, growing by means of the primitive node, constitute a unique organizing cell line of basic morphogenic importance. The cells of the notochordal canal, and later the notochordal plate, provide inducing mechanisms which are decisive in the formation of neuroectoderm (brain and medullary tube). After formation and closure of the neural tube, the notochordal plate separates from neural tissue and, as the notochord, becomes the principal organizing structure of the spine, attracting (sclerotomal) mesenchyme to form the spine. The notochordal cells first induce the formation and organization of the neural tube and, after fulfilling this task, organize the formation of the vertebrae.

During the period of early neural induction (early neurulation), the notochordal plate adheres to the overlying ectoderm. During the second half of the 3rd week of development, the ectoderm adjacent to the notochordal plate, which constitutes a distinct rostrocaudal axis of the now 2-mm embryo, thickens and forms the neural groove.

Related to the neurulation process, the elevated embryo separates from the surface of the amniotic sac, the early morphogenesis of the heart becomes evident, and the dorsal intraembryonic portion of the yolk sac becomes incorporated into the embryonic body. A narrow channel growing from the yolk sac into the connecting stalk, anterior to the cloacal membrane, is known as the allantois. The conceptus consists of three vesicles (Figure 3.11).

CHAPTER 4

The external form of the embryo: organogenesis, formation of somites, late neurulation and the cylindrical embryo

At the end of blastogenesis, the cellular material for constituting the embryo consists of ectoderm, endoderm and mesoderm, and the main organizing structure is the notochordal plate. (In addition, there are primordial germ cells, which do not participate in the formation of germ layers.) By consensus of anatomists and embryologists, the formation of the somites (Figures 4.1–4.12) is regarded as the beginning of organogenesis. The somites are vesicles constituted from dorsal mesoderm, located on both sides along the closing neural groove. The developmental sequence is as follows. The notochordal plate induces transformation of the overlying ectoderm into the neuroectoderm of the neural groove, creating a dorsal developmental field between the neuroectoderm, surface ectoderm and endoderm. In this field, by means of cell-to-cell interactions, the mesoderm becomes segmented and organized into somites. Somites are formed in the craniocaudal sequence. The border between the neuroectoderm and the surface ectoderm becomes visible, starting at the level of the fourth pair of somites, shortly before the neuroectodermal groove closes into the neural tube; the closure extends in the cranial as well as the caudal direction. Cranially, most of the neuroectoderm of the original germ disk develops into the brain plate. In early-somite embryos, the brain plate develops into the three primary portions of the brain: the forebrain, the midbrain and the hindbrain. The most anterior fold of the forebrain is the primordium of the retina of the eyes. As the neural tube closes, its temporarily open ends are known as the rostral and the caudal neuropores. The rostral neuropore closes on about day 27, and the caudal neuropore closes on about days 28–29. The closing of the neural tube is realized by the dorsal approach of the thickened lateral portions of the neural groove, while growth of the ventral medullary plate adherent to the notochordal plate is inhibited (Figures 4.10 and 4.11).

The neuroepithelium of the neural groove is delineated by apical and basal limiting membranes. As the dorsal portions of both sides of the neural groove approach and meet, the apical limiting membrane closes over the cavity of the neural tube, while the basal limiting membrane of the neuroepithelium remains temporarily incomplete dorsally, leaving an open fissure beneath the surface ectoderm. The neuroectodermal cells migrate into this space and provide the neuroectodermal material of the neural crest. Adjacent to each somite, the cells of the neural crest form a spinal ganglion. Additional neural crest cells migrate, contributing to all organs of the body. Melanocytes, the dark brown pigment-forming cells, as well as odontoblasts, or dentine-forming cells, are derivatives of the neural crest cells.

In total, 38 pairs of somites form along the neural tube in the craniocaudal sequence. The most anterior three pairs of somites dismantle in the field of the rhombencephalic vesicle, and contribute to the mesenchyme of the head. The next eight pairs in the sequence are the cervical somites (the first pair of cervical somites fuses with the base of the occipital bone), then 12 pairs are thoracic somites, five are lumbar, five sacral and five coccygeal. Each somite exhibits a dorsolateral portion, the dermatome, which forms the connective tissue of the skin, and a ventromedially located sclerotome which contributes the mesenchyme of the vertebrae.

After the sclerotomic portion of each somite separates, the remaining portion transforms into the dermatomyotome. A bundle of myoblasts

differentiates on the inner surface of the dermatome; the myotomes give rise to all striated skeletal muscles. The early-somite stage (or stage of late
neurulation) begins with the formation of the first
somites (days 20–21) and ends with the closure of
the posterior neuropore (days 29–30). During this
period, the early development of the most important organs takes place. Complicated inductions are
realized by means of various developmental fields,
and are related to the combinations and interactions of various cell subpopulations. The following
primordia of organs appear: the brain vesicles, reti-
nal (optic) vesicles and otic placodes (internal ear);
the medullary tube, neural crest and spinal ganglia;
the olfactory placodes, inducing the development of
the cerebral hemispheres and nose; pharyngeal
arches and pouches, related to the formation of the
middle and external ear, tongue and some organs
located in the neck; the axial skeleton, the limbs and
myotomes of striated muscles, forming the most
important components of the locomotive system. In
addition, the heart loop beats within the pericardial
cavity and blood corpuscles supplied by the yolk sac
circulate within the main vessels. In relation to
regional differentiation, the endodermal digestive
tube transforms into the segments of foregut,
midgut and hindgut. Trabeculae of liver cells prolif-
erate into the vitelline veins. The pancreatic primordia appear. The respiratory organs, bronchi with
mesenchyme, grow into the pleuroperitoneal cavity.
Following the formation of the celomic cavity, the
differentiation of the retroperitoneal organs begins,
forming the kidneys and gonads.

Early human development during the first 4
weeks of life can be summarized as follows. The
oocyte, the blastomeres and the early blastocyst are
spherical, surrounded by the zona pellucida of the
oocyte. The internal diameter of the space delineated by the zona is about 120 μ. The bilaminar
embryonic disk is flat and round with a diameter (at
the age of 14 days) of 0.2 mm. The trilaminar embryonic disk is pear-shaped, at 20 days approximately
1.5 mm in length and 0.8 mm in width, with a very
distinct axial neural groove. During the 4th week,
the embryo becomes elevated above the bottom of
the amniotic sac, the neural groove closes, and the
intraembryonic endoderm bulges from the yolk sac
within the anterior and posterior portions of the
embryo and transforms into the primitive gut. At
the end of the 4th week, the embryo is 3.5–4 mm in
length, dorsally concave and cylindrical, with
distinct somites.

In relation to the early development of the external form of the embryo, the most important trans-
formations are positional changes of the notochord.
During closure of the neural tube, the notochordal
plate adheres to the neuroectoderm, as well as to
the primordium of the digestive tube. After the closure of the neural tube, the notochordal plate
detaches from both the neural tube and the endoderm of the digestive tube, and transforms into the
notochord (Figures 4.11 and 4.12). During the
24 h following the detachment of the notochordal
plate, the embryo changes its general form from
cylindrical and dorsally concave to a typical
C shape, dorsally convex.

CHAPTER 5

The C-shaped embryo with differentiating limbs

C-shaped embryos exhibit differentiation of limbs (Figures 5.1–5.17). The ventral bending of the head of the embryo is a mechanical consequence of the attachment of the rostral head-end of the notochord to the Rathke's pouch, and the anchoring of the spinal portion of the notochord in the bodies of the vertebrae. The head portion of the notochord is in the position of the string of a bow. As the primordia of the brain grow, the different portions of the brain fold over the blastema of the basal cartilage of the skull. As the prosencephalon is fixed, the midbrain and the terminal portions of the hindbrain are the areas of flexure. Originally, there are three brain vesicles: the forebrain, the midbrain and the hindbrain. The forebrain differentiates into two portions: the diencephalon, located caudal from the stalks of the optic cups, and the telencephalon. Induction of mitotic activity within the telencephalon by olfactory placodes is the principal stimulus needed for the development of the brain hemispheres. The mesencephalon is the flexible tube between the forebrain and the hindbrain. The hindbrain gives rise to the metencephalon and the myelencephalon. These two portions of the brain are related in the embryonic period to the formation of the fourth cerebral ventricle.

Rostral from the vertebral column, the notochord is located ventral to the basal cartilage of the skull. The terminal portion of the myelencephalon bends as the cervical flexure of the brain. Mesencephalic and cervical flexures are dorsally convex; the metencephalic (pontine) flexure is dorsally concave.

The spinal cord extends from the hindbrain along the entire length of the embryo and is supported by the vertebral column, which is formed around the notochord.

The dorsal outline of the embryo depends on the formation of the brain and spinal cord, protected by the skull and vertebral column. The ventral outline of the embryo is related to the formation of the brain, nose, mouth, pharyngeal arches, heart, liver, umbilical cord and external genitalia. The limbs appear laterally on the embryonic body. Their characteristic morphological changes during the embryonic stage, from a simple bud to a trisegmental extremity with fingers or toes, represent a good basis for the determination of embryonic age.

CHAPTER 6

The late embryo and the fetus

The late embryo exhibits definitive human traits (Figures 6.1 and 6.2). The limbs are fully differentiated, including fingers and toes. The difference between the embryo and the fetus is evident. In the embryo, the eye fissures are open, or closing; in the fetus, the eyelids are completely closed. The rims of the eyelids fuse between days 56 and 60 of development.

The fetal face is human in appearance (Figure 6.3). On the fingers and toes, nail plates are distinct. In the early fetus, well-defined volar pads on the fingers and toes precede differentiation of dermal ridges. Depending upon the location of the volar pads, highly individual dermatoglyphic patterns acquire their characteristics.

During the early fetal stage, the skin undergoes marked changes. The embryonic epidermis is a simple ectodermal epithelium, which transforms in late embryos into a bilaminar epithelium known as the periderm. Peridermal cells constitute a characteristic 'pavement' of surface cuboidal cells, full of glycogen. As the peridermal epidermis changes into a cornifying multilayered epidermis, the peridermal cells detach and become suspended within the amniotic fluid. The amniotic fluid is swallowed by the fetus, and the peridermal cells are the first intrauterine food accepted by mouth. Remnants of digested peridermal cells contribute to meconium within the fetal gut.

Hair follicles (primordia of hair) become visible during the early fetal stage. At the mid-fetal stage, the first generation of hair covers the entire body of the fetus, especially the limbs, face and back. The downy coat is termed lanugo. However, lanugo hairs are temporary and disappear during the perinatal period. The next generation of hair developing after birth constitutes the prepubertal hair, known as vellus.

The eyelashes appear at about gestational week 20.

As subcutaneous fat accumulates during the late fetal stage, at mid-gestation the fetal vessels are very prominent.

Finally, during the fetal stage, all organs become functional.

CHAPTER 7

The development of the head and face

It has been provocatively stated in discussions with politicians that the head is formed around the mouth and that the brain and nose are later acquisitions. In fact, the first structure of the future head is the prechordal plate, which is present in trilaminar embryos in front of the notochordal canal. The prechordal plate is the inner layer of the oral buccopharyngeal membrane, which closes for a short time, in early-somite embryos, the entrance into the digestive tube (Figure 7.1). Other structures of the future head are the ectoderm-covered brain vesicles with optic cups, and the first and second pharyngeal arches and pouches located around the ear vesicles and supporting the wall of the primitive pharynx. The pharyngeal arches and pouches are covered externally by ectoderm and internally by endoderm. The paired olfactory placodes induce formation of brain hemispheres and are important 'organizing centers' of the face. The primitive mouth (stomodeum) is a triangular fold delineated by the forebrain with optic cups and by the two first pharyngeal arches (Figure 7.2). The bottom of the fold is provided by the oral membrane, which disintegrates between days 23 and 24, leaving the mouth open, providing an entrance into the anterior gut (the primordium of the pharynx). As the maxillary centers, primordia of the upper jaws, appear laterally on the first pharyngeal arches, the shape of the primitive mouth becomes pentagonal. The first pharyngeal arches fuse into a single mandibular arch, which precedes formation of the lower jaw (Figure 7.3). In addition, the mandibular arch contributes the anterior portion of the tongue, and the lower lip of the mouth. The bottom structures of the primitive oral cavity, including the tongue, are provided by internal portions of the pharyngeal arches.

The formations of the upper lip, upper jaw (maxillae) and nose are closely interrelated. The most important structures in this region are the two olfactory placodes, which originate from accumulation of neuroectodermal olfactory cells. The placodes are located laterally, anterior to the developing eyes, on the rim of the oral cavity (Figure 7.4). The olfactory placodes attract mesenchyme of the pharyngeal arches, located originally behind the eyes. This material develops from the second pharyngeal arch to the olfactory placodes as oculonasal mesenchyme, and forms a nasal ridge around each placode. Each nasal ridge has premaxillary and medial and lateral nasal portions. Horseshoe-shaped nasal ridges transform the olfactory placodes into nasal pits (Figures 7.5 and 7.6). The maxillary primordium is temporarily separated from the lateral portion of the oculonasal mesenchyme by a deep nasolacrimal furrow, and, between the maxillary primordium and the premaxillary portion of the nasal ridge, there exists a temporary epithelial plate of the lip (Figures 7.7–7.9). The epithelial plates disappear as the mesenchymal maxillary and premaxillary primordia fuse. Failure of the premaxillary and maxillary primordia to fuse results in a cleft lip. The most anterior extension of the axial skeleton is the prechordal mesenchyme, which contributes the nasal capsule including the nasal septum. The most anterior portion of the nasal capsule makes the tip of the nose. The prechordal mesenchyme 'glues' the medial portions of both nasal ridges together, and its superficial portion is involved in the formation of the philtrum of the upper lip. The superficial mesenchyme, in the vicinity of the corners of the inner eye, covers the nasolacrimal sulcus and provides the mesenchyme of the upper cheeks (Figures 7.10–7.12). The craniofacial development is often affected by malformations (Figures 7.13–7.15).

CHAPTER 8

The skeleton and striated muscles

The skeleton originates from mesenchyme, which is the embryonic connective tissue that fills the spaces between epithelial structures. The first generation of intraembryonic desmogenic mesenchyme is derived mainly from the sclerotomes of early somites, and from somatopleure and splanchnopleure. The cartilaginous primordia originate from mesenchymal condensations known as blastemas. The blastemas of vertebrae are derived from the second generation of cells proliferating from sclerotomes which have detached from somites. Within the vertebral blastemas, the positions of the original somites are occupied by spinal ganglia, and the somites transform into dermatomyotomes. The separated sclerotomes are disposed ventrolaterally in the spaces between the spinal ganglia, in the intersegmental position. Streams of the chondrogenic second generation of sclerotomic mesenchymal cells accumulate around the notochord, detached from the medullary tube and from the gut, and provide the cartilaginous vertebral bodies, while the primary desmogenic generation of sclerotomic mesenchyme remains located in the caudal half of each segment, as primordia of the intervertebral disks. At this stage, characterized by early differentiation of hand and foot plates of limbs, human embryos exhibit temporally a double dorsal segmentation, related to both the formation of the vertebrae by the sclerotomes, and the presence of the spinal ganglia in place of the early somites.

The cartilaginous axial skeleton of the head and body consists of the skull, vertebral column, ribs and sternum. The bones of the limbs include, on the upper limb, the clavicle, the scapula, the humerus, the ulna and radius, the carpal and metacarpal bones, and the phalanges of the fingers, and, on the lower limb, the lateral pelvic bones (ilium, pubis and ischium), the femur, the tibia, the fibula, the tarsus and metatarsus, and the phalanges of the toes (Figures 8.1–8.17).

The development of the bones starts from condensed mesenchyme (blastema) providing cartilaginous models of each bone (Figures 8.18–8.21). The gene determination of this marvellous structural differentiation is completely unknown. The mesenchyme around cartilages forms the perichondrium, which connects neighboring cartilaginous models of bones separated by spaces filled with loose mesenchyme. As the fluid appears between bones within the cavities of future joints, these joints are established and the surrounding mesenchyme contributes the joint capsules.

The cartilaginous models are replaced by bones via perichondral and endochondral ossification. Perichondral ossification is characterized by the deposition of compact sheets of bone tissue on the surface of the cartilage. Endochondral ossification begins with the hypertrophy and calcification of cartilaginous cells inside the cartilaginous model of bone. Then, osteoclasts and osteoblasts from the perichondrium invade the hypertrophied cartilage. Osteoclasts dissolve the cartilage and, simultaneously, osteoblasts form spongy trabeculae of bone material. Osteoblasts synthesize osteoid, the extracellular material necessary for the deposition of hydroxyapatite crystals (calcium-containing bone mineral). The areas of ossifying trabeculae inside the cartilaginous models of bones are known as the ossifying centers (Figures 8.22–8.24).

Ossification of the flat bones of the skull is desmogenic, not preceded by cartilages (Figure 8.25).

Morphogenesis of the limbs begins in the lateral mesodermal plate of the embryo on about days

30–35, by accumulation of special ectodermal cells. As the mesenchymal cells underneath multiply, the region develops into the beginnings of a limb bud. The special ectodermal cells become concentrated to form the apical ectodermal ridge. Under the apical ectodermal ridge, endothelial cells form the venous marginal sinus and a plexus of capillaries within the limb plate. The ectodermal apical ridge provides growth factors, and is probably involved in the resorption of nutrients from the amniotic fluid. The apical ectodermal ridge represents a 'nutritive structure' related to the general growth of the limb, not to its differentiation. After days 35–38, the arterial primordia, myoblasts and the nerve trunks develop into the limb buds. A zone of polarizing activity is located at the distal end of the ectodermal apical ridge, and this controls the formation of the digits or toes. The cartilaginous skeleton appears in a proximo–distal sequence, from the brachial girdle to the humerus to the fingers, and from the pelvic girdle to the femur to the toes. The limbs are covered by ectoderm, which gives rise to the epidermis of the skin. The segmental origin of the dermis is evident from the sensitive segmental innervation provided by neurons located in adjacent spinal ganglia. The bones, preceded by cartilages, are formed by the mesenchyme of the limb buds and by cells immigrating into the region via the vessels. The skeletal muscles originate from the myotomes of adjacent segments. Tendons are connected with the periosteum; if the typical area of insertion is not present, they locate in the neighborhood of the bone, connective tissue or another tendon. If the muscle does not reach the tendon, the tendon degenerates and disappears. The motor innervation of the muscles is provided by neurons located in the medullary tube, in the medullary segment adjacent to the myotome involved in the formation of the muscle.

CHAPTER 9

The vessels, the heart and circulation of the blood

The vessels

The primordia of the main vessels appear as endothelial tubes long before the blood circulates. The endothelium (lining of vessels) and blood corpuscles originate from a common precursor cell, the endotheliohemocytoblast. First hemocytoblasts are provided by cells of the primary mesoderm in the wall of the yolk sac. The blood is a suspension of blood corpuscles within a protein-containing fluid, the blood plasma. The blood circulates within vessels; the heart pumps blood into the arteries which carry it to all organs and tissues. Capillary networks within the tissues are sites of metabolic exchange between the blood and the cells of the organs. The interstitial fluid is filtered back from the tissues into the venous capillaries. The veins then carry the blood from the capillaries to the heart.

Within the embryo, there are three distinct blood circulatory systems. The first is the vitelline circulation, which transports the blood corpuscles formed on the yolk sac into the embryo. As the heart begins beating (on about days 22–24), blood flows from the aortopulmonary segment of the heart loop, by way of the third aortic arches, to the head and through the fourth, left aortic arch into the descending aorta. Some of the visceral branches of the descending aorta enter the capillary network around blood islands on the yolk sac. Corpuscles formed and released by the blood islands of the yolk sac enter the blood and return to the sinus of the heart loop via vitelline veins. This vitelline circulation is temporary, as the blood-forming capacity of the yolk sac becomes exhausted during the 8th week of development.

The second circulatory system is the intraembryonic one supplying blood to embryonic tissues. During the first 4 weeks, all embryonic tissues are nourished by diffusion. The intraembryonic circulation begins during the 5th developmental week, as the aortopulmonary segment of the heart loop, followed by the aorta, receives blood ejected by the primordia of both heart ventricles. From the aorta, the blood flows to the head on the right side by way of the brachiocephalic (innominate) artery and via the common carotid artery on the left side. The upper limbs are supplied with arterial blood by subclavian arteries. The body wall receives blood from parietal branches of the aorta, the organs located retroperitoneally behind the peritoneal cavity (adrenals, kidneys and gonads) from the intermediate branches, and the digestive organs from the visceral branches of the descending aorta. The intraembryonic terminal branches of the aorta provide blood for the pelvic organs and lower limbs.

The third circulatory system involves the two umbilical arteries, which are the main terminal branches of the descending aorta during intrauterine life. Through these arteries, fetal blood enters the placenta, including the capillary networks within the placental villi. There, fetomaternal and maternofetal metabolic exchanges take place. Arterial blood flowing from the embryo into the placenta is deoxygenated and carries metabolic waste, while venous blood, leaving the placenta via placental veins that join to form the single umbilical vein, is oxygenated and rich in nourishing substances. The umbilical vein passes through the fetal liver and enters the inferior vena cava, which collects blood from the caudal portion of the embryonic body, the visceral organs and the legs. From the head, neck and superior extremities, blood returns to the heart by way of the superior vena cava. This third circulatory system is known as the fetoplacental circulation.

The heart

The heart is a pump which moves blood within the vessels. The beating heart loop is the first functioning intraembryonic organ. The first beats or contractions appear between days 22 and 24 in 2.5-mm embryos with a closing neural tube and the first ten somite pairs. The frequency of the early embryonic heartbeat is slow, but increases rapidly, reaching 160 beats/min at the end of the embryonic stage. The heartbeat frequency of a newborn is about 140 beats/min. The embryochorionic circulation becomes established during the 5th developmental week and represents the anatomical constitution of the embryochorionic, and later fetoplacental, unit. After this stage, the embryo is unable to survive without the fetoplacental circulation, and the chorion will not survive without the beating embryonic heart. The beating heart is the most important sign of embryonic viability, and is detectable using ultrasound.

The heart tube

The heart originates from mesoderm contributing myocardial cells and cardiac jelly, epicardial cells and endothelial cells. The endothelial cells provide the lining of endocardium, the innermost component of the heart wall. The sensory innervation of the heart originates from neuroectodermal neurons growing from the neural crest.

The first step in the development of the heart is the formation of the pericardial cavity, which appears within the cephalic mesoderm on about day 20. The mesodermal cells of the epicardial splanchnopleure located close to the midline transform into myocardial cells around a space containing cells derived from the primary mesoderm, originally scattered between germ layers of the germ disk. These endothelial cells differentiate into capillaries, and fuse to a single endocardial tube located within the tube of myocardial cells and cardiac jelly, thus constituting the myoendocardial heart tube. The heart tube is attached caudally to the venous sinus which receives the inflowing veins (cardinal, umbilical and vitelline). At first, venous fluid without blood corpuscles fills the heart tube; the tube becomes distended and reacts by contracting. The heart begins to beat in response to filling (Figures 9.1–9.4).

Heart loop segmentation, septation and valves

As the heart tube elongates and its inflow and outflow ends converge, it bends into an asymmetrical conformation within the embryo. The human heart loop is convex to the right side, and the myocardium forms a 'basket' on the convexity. On the loop, the primordia of both ventricles share a common myocardial basket. Between both ventricles, on the concave portion of the loop, there is a distinct interventricular incisure. The efflux portion of the loop is characterized by a thick, glucosaminoglycan subendothelial layer. After formation of the loop, the process of coiling of the loop is described as wedging. The wedging brings the two ventricular portions of the loop together, and the bulbus of the heart becomes placed anterior to both ventricles. The left ventricle becomes continuous with both the right ventricle and the bulbus of the loop. Simultaneously with wedging, septation of the heart becomes evident. The inflow (atrial) segment of the heart bulges to the left and right sides, forming the auricles of the atria. At the end of wedging, between the atria and both ventricles, there is a distinct spiral inflow ring located above the opening of the right and below the opening of the left atrium. At this stage, the end of the 5th week of development, the interatrial, atrioventricular and aortopulmonary septation begins. The muscular interventricular septum is distinct. Septation takes about 14 days to be completed. During this period, the right and left atria become separated by two interatrial folds: the membranous septum primum and the fleshy septum secundum. The common atrioventricular opening of the heart tube becomes divided into the right and left atrioventricular openings. Coincidentally, within the right atrioventricular opening, the tricuspid valve becomes evident, while around the left atrioventricular opening the bicuspid (mitral) valve is formed. Right and left ventricles are separated by the muscular portion of the interventricular septum, and by a small membranous portion of the interventricular septum located close to the atrioventricular valves. The right ventricle separates from the rest of the bulbus, which represents the aortopulmonary segment. Septation of the aortopulmonary segment by two spiral aortopulmonary ridges gives rise to the septum, which separates the ascending portions of the aorta and of the pulmonary artery. The pulmonary artery opens into the right ventricle; the aorta opens into the left ventricle. The small membranous portion of the interventricular septum contains connective tissue located between the pulmonary artery and the ring of the mitral valve (Figures 9.5–9.8).

The epicardium and coronary vessels

The early myocardium is a special muscular tissue with distinct channels that facilitate the diffusion of nourishing substances from the cavity of the heart tube (Figures 9.9 and 9.10). Very early, during the 6th week, a capillary network is formed within the epicardium. Mesothelial cells and fibroblasts of the epicardium spread on the myoendocardial tube from the site of attachment of the heart tube to the pericardial wall by mesocardium. During the 6th week, a venous capillary network is formed in the subepicardial region, draining fluid into the coronary veins. Beginning at the 7th week, ingrowth of the coronary arteries from the aorta connects the coronary capillaries and veins with the arterial bloodstream, establishing the coronary circulation. In many embryonic organs, the development of vessels follows the same pattern: first appears the capillary network and draining veins are formed (vasculogenesis); then follows the ingrowth of the arteries (angiogenesis). Angiogenesis of coronary arteries starts the coronary circulation within the organ (Figures 9.11–9.17).

The fetal blood circulation

During the fetal stage, blood from the caudal portion of the body and legs returns to the heart by way of the inferior vena cava. This blood is deoxygenated (venous). However, before reaching the heart, behind the liver, the inferior vena cava receives oxygenated blood from the umbilical vein coming from the placenta.

The superior vena cava carries deoxygenated blood from the head and upper extremities. Within the right atrium there is a mixture, of which two-thirds is oxygenated and one-third is deoxygenated blood. From the right atrium, there are two blood-streams: one goes to the right ventricle and into the pulmonary artery, and the other flows to the left atrium through the open foramen ovale between the atrial septa. The fetal main pulmonary artery transports a substantial amount of blood via a large shunt, the arterial duct (duct of Botallus), into the aorta, while the proper pulmonary arteries receive just a little blood supplying the non-functioning lungs. The blood from the right atrium, entering the left atrium by the open interatrial foramen ovale, mixes with a small amount of deoxygenated blood returning to the left atrium by way of the pulmonary veins, enters the left heart ventricle through the left atrioventricular opening, and is ejected into the aorta. Within the descending aorta, the blood from the aortic arch mixes with the blood shunted by the arterial duct. During intrauterine life, all fetal tissues are supplied with incompletely oxygenated blood.

After birth, there is sudden circulatory turmoil as the placenta is rejected and respiration begins. Clamping or tightening of the umbilical cord terminates the placental circulation, while the onset of breathing opens the cardiopulmonary circulation. As the blood pressure in the left heart atrium increases, the interatrial septum closes, preventing the interatrial stream of blood. The arterial duct is obliterated during the first days of extrauterine life; the shunting of blood from the pulmonary artery into the aorta becomes impossible. Consequently, after birth, the venous (deoxygenated) blood, from all tissues except the lungs, enters the right atrium via the superior and inferior vena cava. Venous blood from the right atrium passes to the right ventricle and to the pulmonary artery; hence, the pulmonary artery contains venous blood. Within the lungs, atmospheric oxygen is absorbed as a result of gaseous exchange between air and hemoglobin in red blood cells and the blood becomes oxygenated. Oxygenated blood from the lungs goes to the heart by way of the pulmonary veins; hence, the pulmonary veins contain arterial blood. This blood enters the left atrium, passes to the left ventricle and is ejected into the aorta. After birth, the arteries, which are branches of the aorta, supply all organs of the body with fully oxygenated blood.

CHAPTER 10

Sex determination: boy or girl

Sex is determined at fertilization: 50% of spermatozoa bear the Y chromosome and 50% of spermatozoa bear the X chromosome. The spermatozoon is haploid with a total of 23 chromosomes. The oocyte, after the second meiotic division is completed, also has a haploid set of 23 chromosomes, but these always include the X chromosome. Consequently, the chromosomal constitution of diploid cells originating from the fertilized oocyte is either 46,XY or 46,XX. As the male sex-determining gene (known as the sex-determining region Y or SRY) is located on the Y chromosome, the chromosomal combination 46,XY determines the male, and is related to testicular differentiation. The chromosomal combination 46,XX, the presence of two X chromosomes in the absence of the Y chromosome, is related to ovarian differentiation, and determines the female.

Primordial germ cells

In vertebrates, including the human, life passes from generation to generation via the sex cells, i.e. spermatozoa in the male and the oocytes in the female. All sex cells are derivatives of primordial germ cells, which represent a special cell line programmed very early within the inner cell mass of the blastocyst. Germ cells do not participate in the differentiation of germ layers (Figure 10.1). In early bilaminar embryos, primordial germ cells are located within the ectoderm of the amniotic sac behind the germ disk. From this region, they migrate into the connective stalk (during formation of the secondary yolk sac) and colonize the endoderm of the hindgut. Subsequently, they migrate through the mesentery into the primordia of the gonads, which are located on the medial side of the urogenital ridges (longitudinal folds bulging into the peritoneal cavity on both sides of the

mesentery). The SRY gene of the Y chromosome triggers a chain of other genes: the genetic cascade of male differentiation, which involves development of the testes, and is followed by differentiation of the male genital ducts and differentiation of the external genitalia.

The basic developmental sequence of primordial germ cells is, first, mitotic proliferation and, second, terminal differentiation coupled with two meiotic divisions. The two meiotic divisions reduce the original two sets of chromosomes of the germ cells into a single chromosomal set. Each mature germ cell exhibits a unique combination of genes mixed from both paternal and maternal chromosomal sets.

Testicular development

The basic difference between the male and female sexes concerns the mitotic developmental sequence of the sex stem cells, the male spermatogonia and the female oogonia. In males, the mitotic proliferation of germ cells (spermatogonia) is preserved throughout life, while, in females, the mitotic capacity of the germ cells (oogonia) is exhausted by their intensive proliferation during fetal life.

In male differentiation, the first changes in the developmental sequence of male primordial germ cells appear at the beginning of gonadal differentiation. These changes, related to their lifelong proliferation, precede the differentiation of the gonadal primordia (gonadal ridges) into testes. Within the testes, the germinal compartment is organized into seminiferous cords containing germinal stem cells, known as spermatogonia, and supportive cells, known as Sertoli cells. The Sertoli cells constitute the cords, and synthesize (starting in the 7th week of development) the anti-Müllerian hormone (AMH), which suppresses the Müllerian ducts. Starting in the 9th week, interstitial cells of the testes (Leydig cells) produce the most important male sex hormone, testosterone. Testosterone and its receptor are the main factors in the growth of the male sexual ducts and differentiation of the male external genitalia.

Ovarian development

Transformation of the gonadal primordia into the ovaries is characterized by extensive mitotic proliferation of germ cells, which exhausts during fetal life their entire capacity to divide mitotically. Prenatally, within the fetal ovaries, the germ cells or oogonia immediately enter their terminal differentiation into oocytes. Still prenatally, the ooctyes undergo the prophase of the first meiotic division, which is the most important step regarding the mixing of paternal and maternal genes. Thereafter, the oocytes are incorporated into the ovarian follicles. Only those oocytes within the follicles can survive the pause between the prophase and metaphase of the first meiotic division, i.e. until ovulation, which extends for the following 12–50 years. Repeated ovulations are characteristic of the fertile period of a woman's life.

There are 4–6 million oocytes formed in each fetal ovary; two million ovarian follicles are present in each ovary of a newborn girl. At 18 years of age, there are 180–200 thousand follicles in each ovary. During the fertile period of a woman's life, about 400 follicles ovulate; the rest degenerate. In women over 60 years of age, no oocytes remain; this period of a woman's life is known as the postmenopause.

Genital ducts

Two pairs of ducts are present in every embryo, regardless of chromosomal sex. These are the meso-

nephric ducts (Wolffian ducts, primary ureters) and the paramesonephric (Müllerian) ducts (Figure 10.2). Both ducts run retroperitoneally and craniocaudally. The mesonephric ducts enter the cloaca. Formation of the Wolffian ducts precedes formation of the Müllerian ducts, which grow in contact with the Wolffian ducts. Caudal to the gonads, the Müllerian ducts cross the Wolffian ducts ventrally, and run parallel near the midline to the urogenital sinus, a derivative of the hindgut (cloaca). The midline, parallel caudal portions of the Müllerian ducts fuse into the uterovaginal canal, a common primordium of the uterus and vagina (Figure 10.3). In males, as a result of the production of AMH and the presence of a specific receptor of AMH in target tissues, the Müllerian ducts regress. AMH reaches the ipsilateral Müllerian ducts by diffusion; regression is limited to the side of the testis that produces the AMH. Consequently, in normal males with bilateral testes, both paramesonephric ducts disappear, apart from some vestigial structures remaining from their most cranial and caudal ends (appendix of the testis, utriculus in the prostate). In contrast to the Müllerian ducts, the growth of the Wolffian ducts is androgen-dependent and requires the presence of testosterone and its receptor. In males, the Wolffian duct changes into the epididymis; the vas deferens is the ejaculatory duct.

In females, no AMH is formed prenatally. Hence, the Müllerian ducts transform into oviducts and into the uterus and most of the vagina. As no testosterone is formed by fetal ovaries, the Wolffian ducts, whose growth is testosterone-dependent, disintegrate, leaving vestigal tubules in the vicinity of the ovaries and oviducts.

External genitalia

In both sexes, the primordia of the external genitalia are the same, originating from structures located around the cloacal membrane. This membrane closes the cloaca, a blind terminal portion of the hindgut. The genital tubercle is an elevated area around the cloacal membrane, anterior to the tail of the embryo; lateral to the genital tubercle are the labioscrotal folds (one on each side) (Figures 10.4–10.7). At the end of the 7th developmental week, as the cloaca is divided by the urorectal septum into the rectum dorsally and the urogenital sinus ventrally, the cloacal membrane splits into the genital membrane, closing the urogenital sinus, and the anal membrane, closing the rectum. The genital membrane disintegrates and disappears in 48–50-day-old embryos; the anal membrane fades approximately 2 days later. Subsequently, as the urogenital sinus opens, the derivative of the genital tubercle is designated as the phallus. The phallus undergoes a sex-related dimorphic differentiation.

Male differentiation (Figures 10.8–10.10) is regulated by testosterone-dependent proteosynthesis. Testosterone in target tissues of the external genitalia is first reduced to dihydrotestosterone, and then bound to a specific receptor protein encoded by a gene located on the X chromosome. The specific testosterone-dependent morphogenic 'male'

steps are formation of the scrotum and closure of the spongy urethra. The labioscrotal folds fuse into the scrotum, and the phallus changes into a penis. The characteristic raphe unifying the scrotum and spongy penile urethra closes in a zipper-like fashion from the rectum to the rim of the glans of the penis.

In females, the growth of the phallus in the absence of testosterone is very limited. The labioscrotal swellings fail to extend to the space anterior to the rectum, and the rims of the urethral groove fail to fuse. The phallus bends ventrally and becomes the clitoris. At the end of the second trimester of pregnancy, in connection with vaginal development, the distance between the clitoris and anus increases, and the rims of the urethral groove are converted into the labia minora, and the labioscrotal folds into the labia majora of the female external genitalia (Figures 10.11–10.14). Prenatally, the ovaries do not influence the development of the female external genitalia or the female genital ducts, i.e. the oviducts, uterus and vagina. Feminine development of the genital ducts and external genitalia occurs in the absence of AMH and testosterone (absence of testes).

SECTION TWO

The human embryo and
fetus illustrated

LIST OF ILLUSTRATIONS

CHAPTER 5

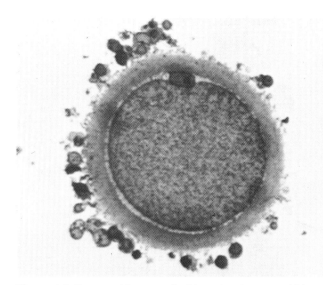

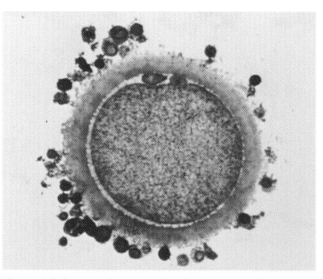

Figure 1.1 Oocyte with zona pellucida: under the zona, within the perivitelline space, the first polar body can be seen. At this stage, the oocyte is released from the ovary

Figure 1.2 Section of oocyte with a detaching second polar body, suggesting completion of second meiotic division

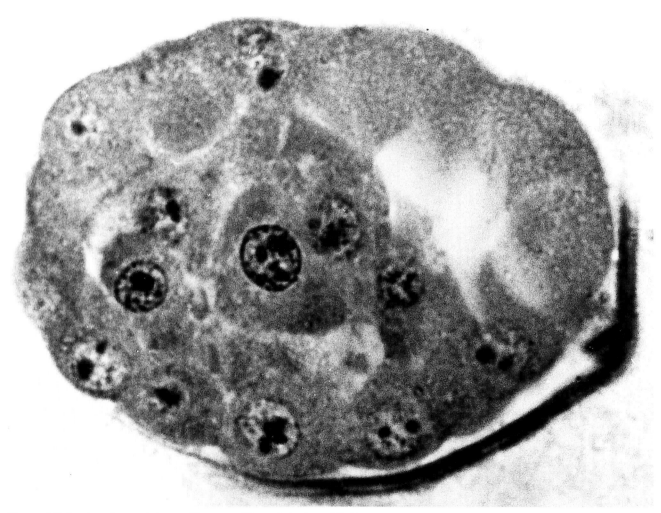

Figure 1.3 Section of an early human blastocyst (Carnegie Institute, Washington, specimen no. 8974; author's micrograph, courtesy of Professor R. O'Rahilly)

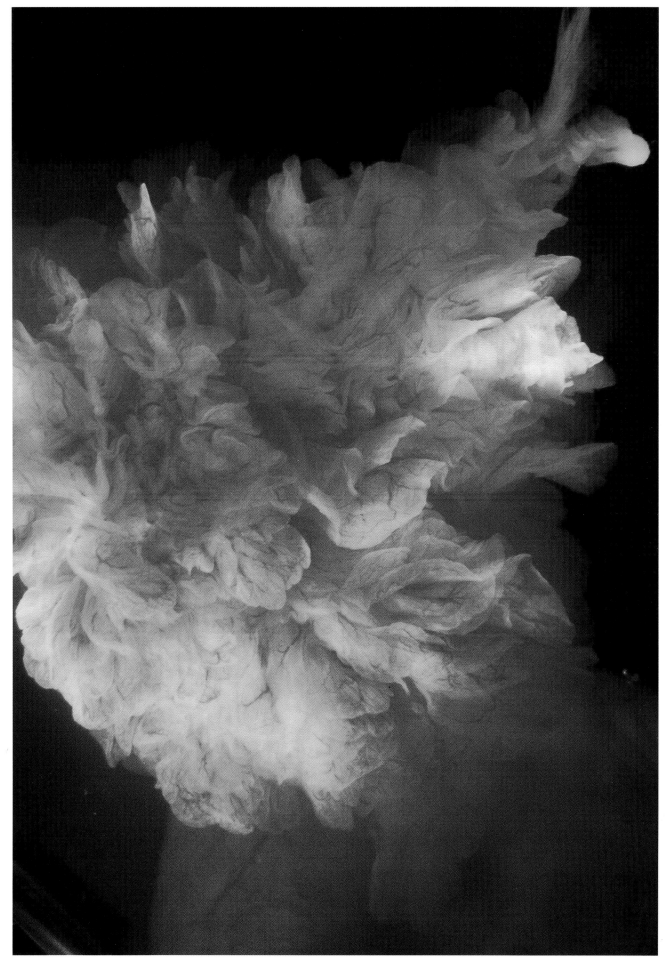

Figure 1.4 Abdominal fimbriated end of the oviduct: the fertilized oocyte enters into its opening and is transported to the uterus

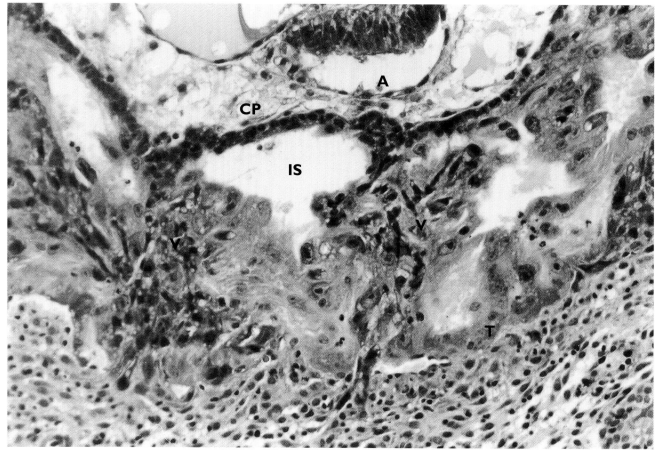

Figure 2.1 Microscopic section of the trophoblastic shell of a 13.5-day-old blastocyst: the shell consists of a chorionic plate (CP), primary chorionic villi (V) separated by primordia of the intervillous space (IS), and peripheral trophoblast (T) growing into the uterine mucosa

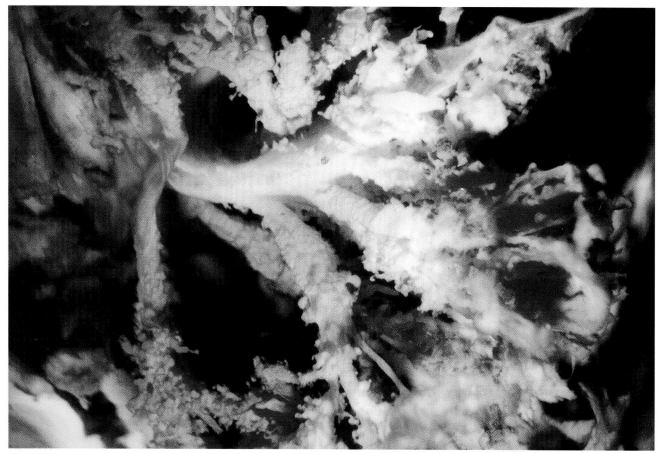

Figure 2.2 Chorionic villi of a 24-day-old embryo

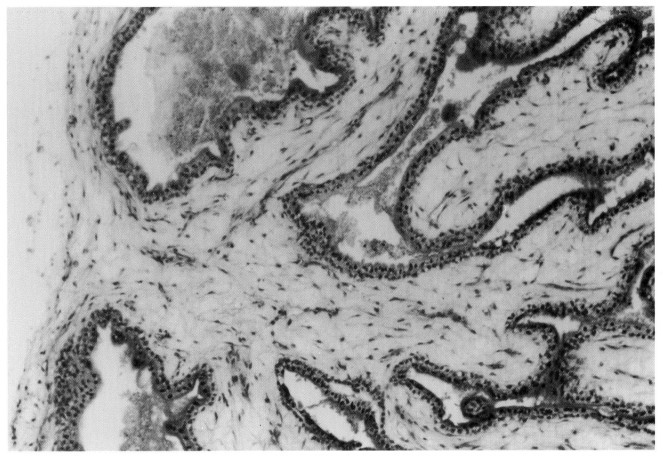

Figure 2.3 Branching chorionic villi of a 22-day-old embryo

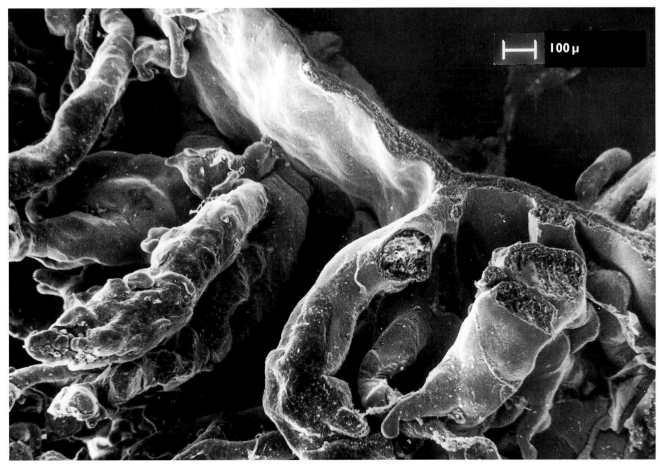

Figure 2.4 Scanning electron micrograph of early chorionic plate and villi

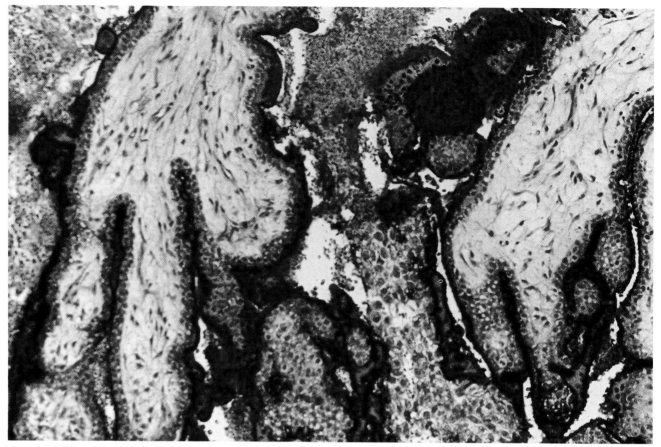

Figure 2.5 Microscopic section of branching chorionic villi: the villi are covered by trophoblast.
Within the mesenchymal stroma can be seen primordia of vessels (22-day-old conceptus).
Maternal blood (yellow) is present within the intervillous space

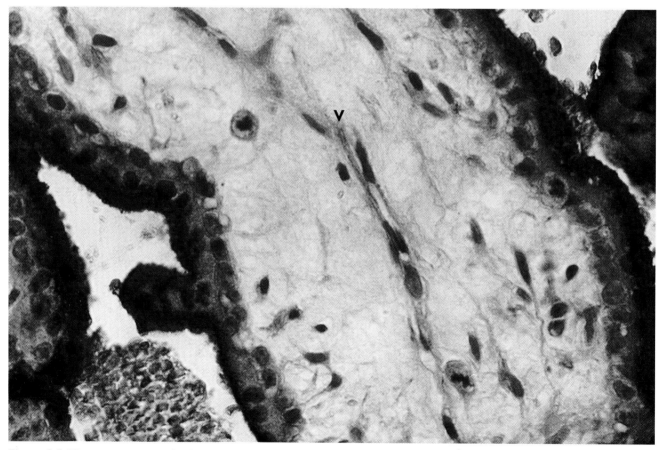

Figure 2.6 Microscopic section of a chorionic villus: the red stain on the surface reflects the
activity of placental alkaline phosphatase; the surface of the villus is covered by trophoblast.
Primordia of vessels (V) are located within the mesenchymal stroma

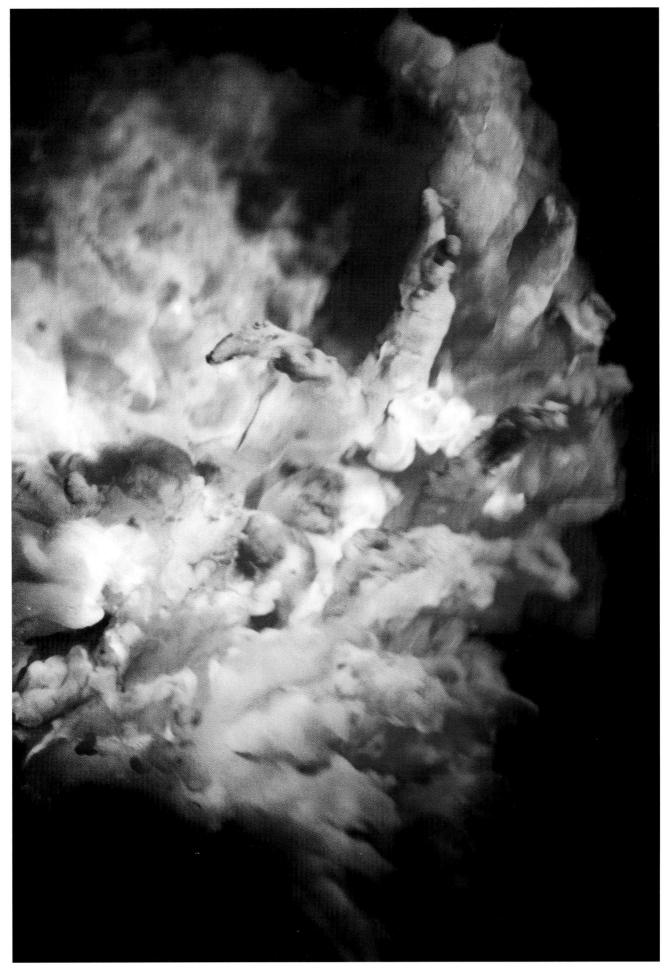

Figure 2.7 Peripheral portion of early chorion

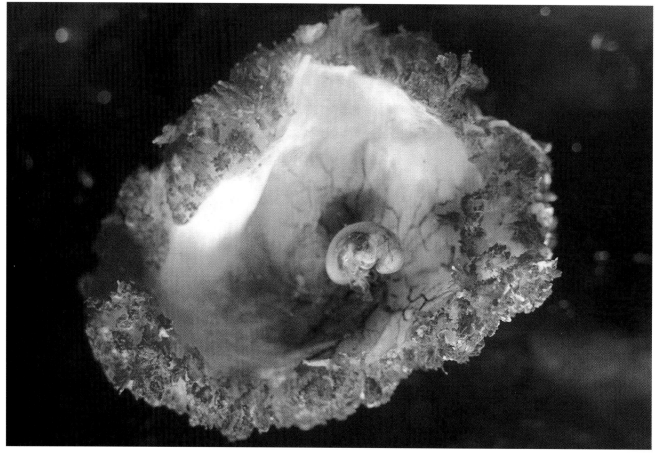

Figure 2.8 A 35-day-old conceptus: the villous chorion. The embryonic vessels bringing blood into the chorion appear black

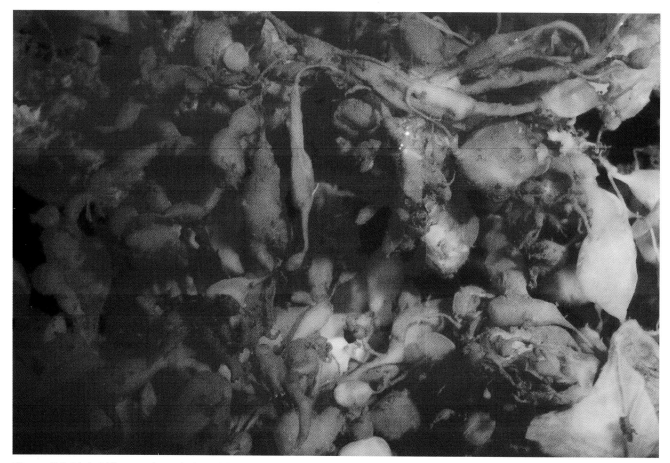

Figure 2.9 Hydatidiform mole: pathological degeneration of chorionic villi, which are avascular and are distended by accumulated fluid

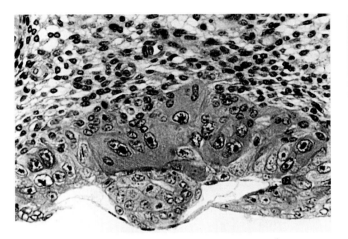

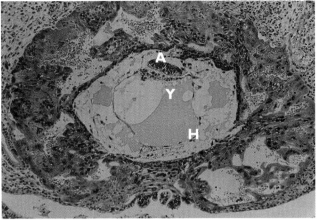

Figure 3.1 Microscopic section of an implanting human blastocyst (day 7) shows invasion of trophoblastic shell into the uterine mucous membrane. The differentiation of the inner cell mass is related to the polarization of cells and formation of basal membranes (Carnegie Institute, Washington, specimen no. 8020; author's micrograph, courtesy of Professor R. O'Rahilly)

Figure 3.2 A 13.5-day-old implanted blastocyst with trophoblastic shell: two apposed vesicles are present, the amniotic sac (A) attached to the trophoblastic shell and the primary yolk sac (Y) delineated by thin cells of Heuser's membrane (H). The area between the two vesicles is the bilaminar germ disk. The ectodermal epithelium of the disk is pseudostratified and cylindrical. The endodermal epithelium is single-layered, exhibiting a craniocaudal gradient in relation to the size of the cells. The endodermal cells are larger at the rostral end of the disk

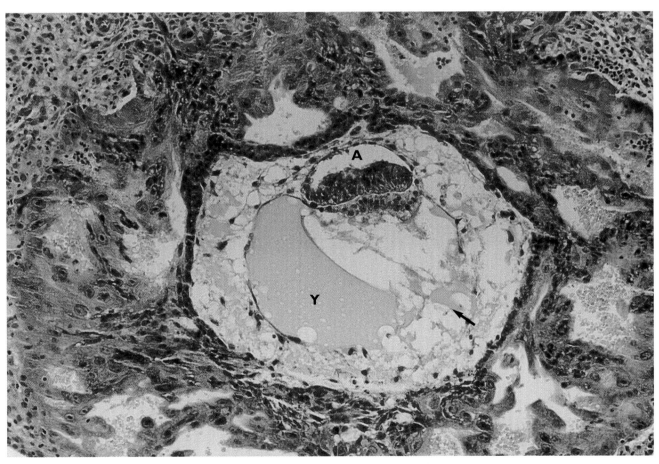

Figure 3.3 Disintegrating primary yolk sac of bilaminar embryo: the yolk sac is filled with a protein-rich 'colloid-like' fluid. As the Heuser's membrane of the primary yolk sac fades (arrow), the content of the sac mixes with extracellular material of the primary mesoderm (only known micrograph of a specimen exhibiting this developmental stage). (A – Amniotic sac, Y – content of primary yolk sac)

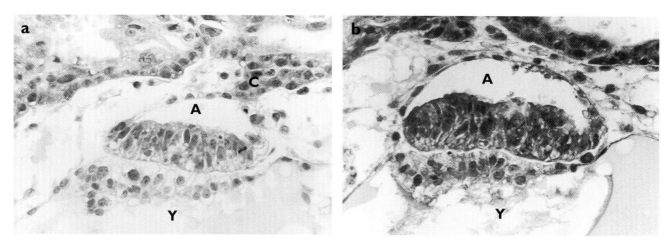

Figure 3.4 Bilaminar embryonic disk of a 13.5-day-old embryo: (a) the amniotic sac (A) is attached to the trophoblastic shell by cytotrophoblastic cells (C); (b) glycogen stain

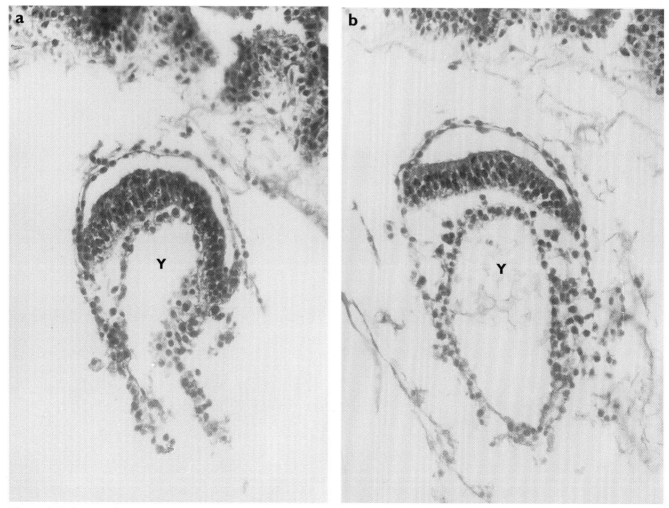

Figure 3.5 Closing of secondary yolk sac, day 15: (a) microscopic section of a bilaminar embryo with an open portion of the yolk sac (Y). (b) Microscopic section of the same embryo with an already closed secondary yolk sac (Y)

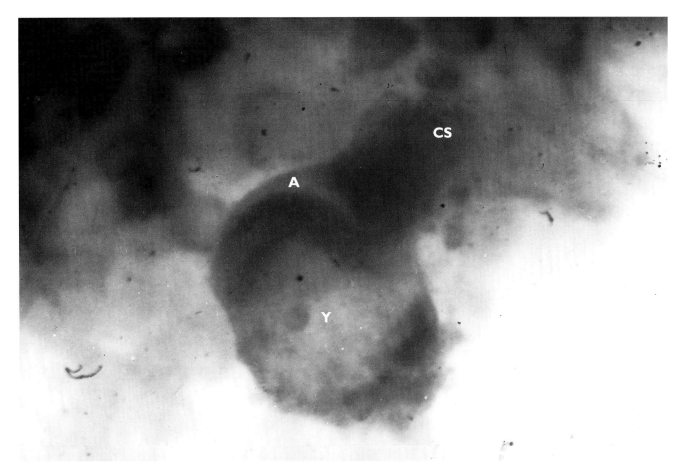

Figure 3.6 Early 16-day-old trilaminar embryo: note two adjacent vesicles attached by a connecting stalk (CS) to the chorion. The embryonic disk is dorsally convex (A – amniotic sac, Y – yolk sac)

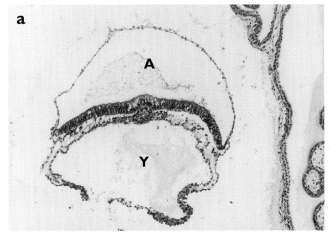

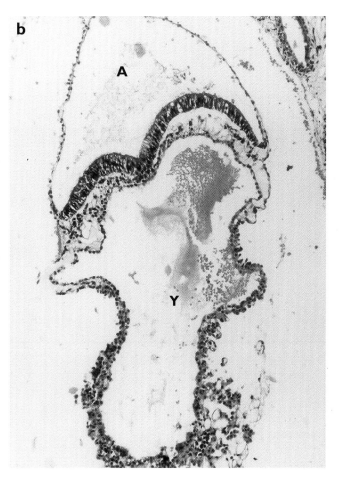

Figure 3.7 Microscopic cross-sections of the embryo shown in Figure 3.6: the area of the embryonic disk is located between the amniotic sac (A) and the yolk sac (Y). Scattered cells of primary mesoderm are present between the ectoderm and the endoderm of the germ disk: (a) cross-section of the notochordal canal anterior to Hensen's node; (b) cross-section of the neural folds of a future cerebral vesicle

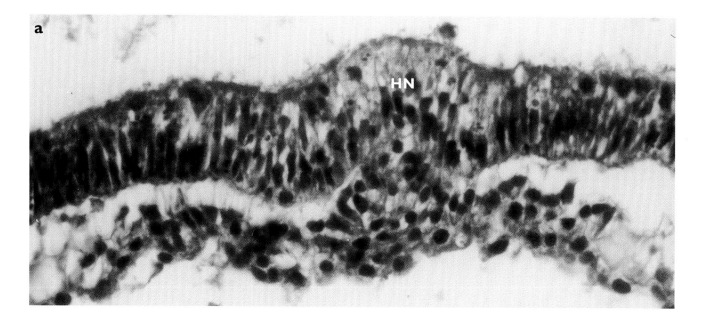

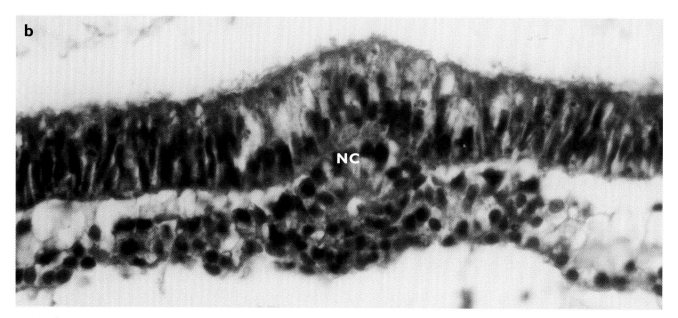

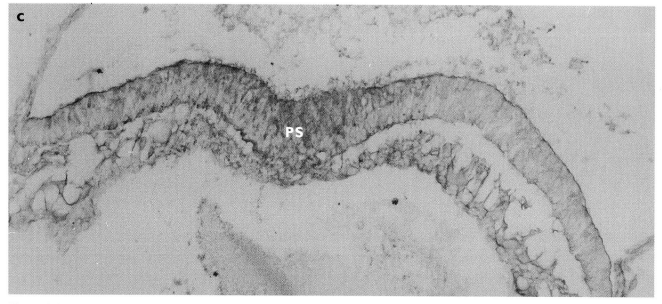

Figure 3.8 Three microscopic sections illustrating the formation of the axial structures of the embryo: (a) Hensen's node (HN) growing from the ectoderm represents the growth center of the notochord; (b) notochordal canal (NC) apposed to the endoderm; (c) early primitive streak (PS) (growth center of the embryonic mesoderm)

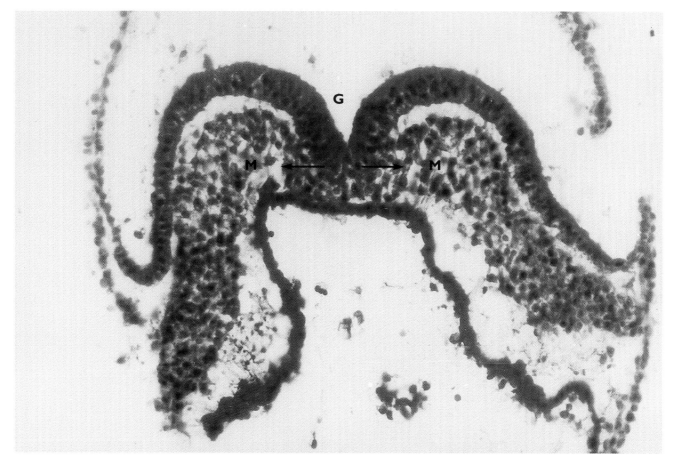

Figure 3.9 Proliferation of mesoderm (M) from the primitive groove (G)

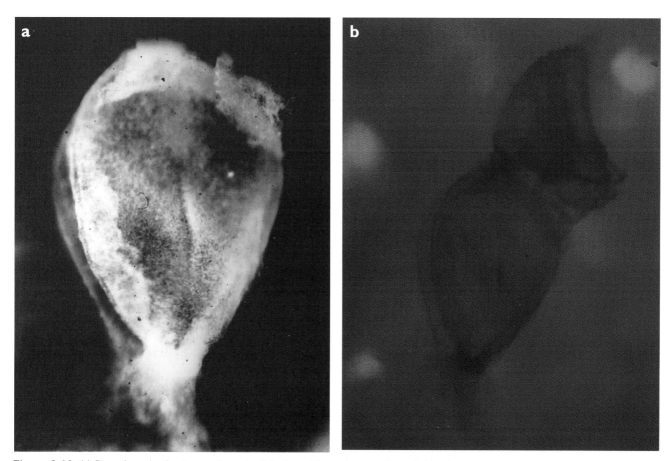

Figure 3.10 (a) Pear-shaped trilaminar embryonic disk viewed from the endodermal side: the yolk sac has been removed (17–18-day-old conceptus). The primitive groove is evident; the allantois extending into the connecting stalk is indistinct; (b) color image of the same embryo

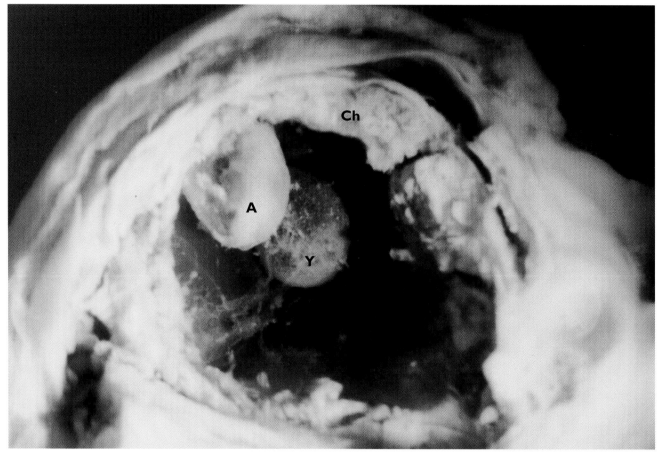

Figure 3.11 Three vesicles representing the implanted conceptus: dissected chorionic sac (Ch) with adjacent amniotic sac (A) and yolk sac (Y)

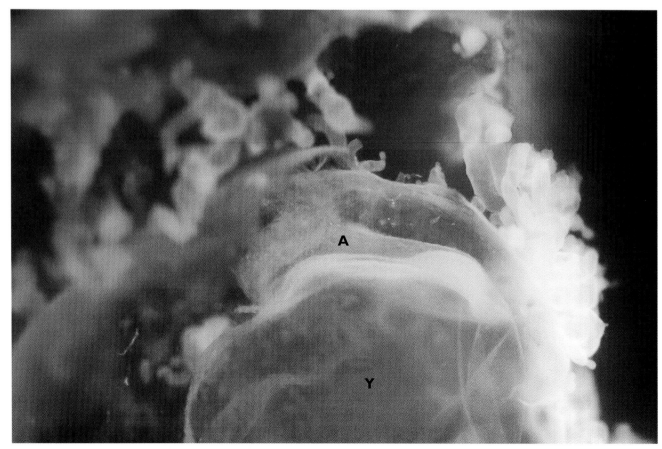

Figure 4.1 Lateral view of a 20-day-old (2 mm) embryo: on the surface can be seen a chorionic plate with villi; the amnion is attached to the chorion by a connecting stalk. The embryo is located within the amniotic sac (A) on the yolk sac (Y). The head is on the right

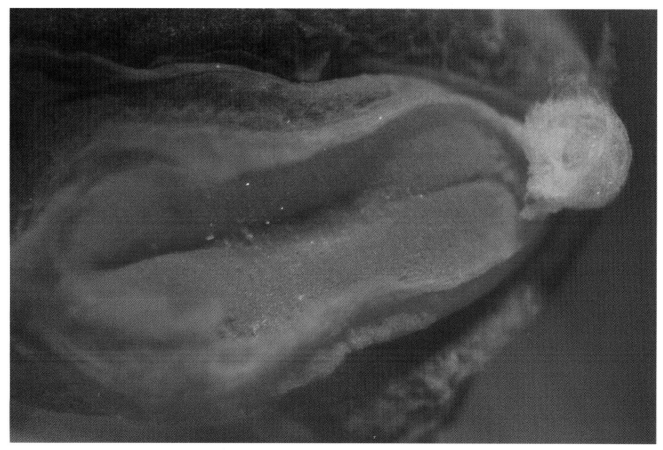

Figure 4.2 Dorsal view of the same embryo shown in Figure 4.1: the brain primordium is divided by a deep and narrow axial furrow. In the middle portion of the embryo, the furrow of the neural groove is broader. In the caudal portion of the embryo, the narrow axial depression is the primitive groove

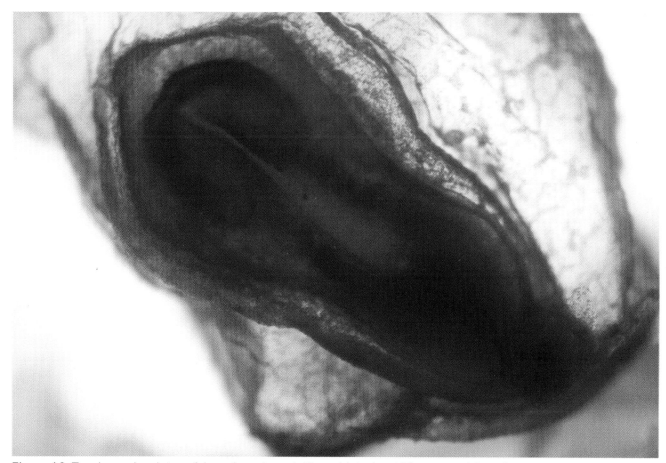

Figure 4.3 Translucent dorsal view of the embryo shown in Figure 4.1: in the middle portion of the embryo can be seen three pairs of differentiating, not yet delineated, somites

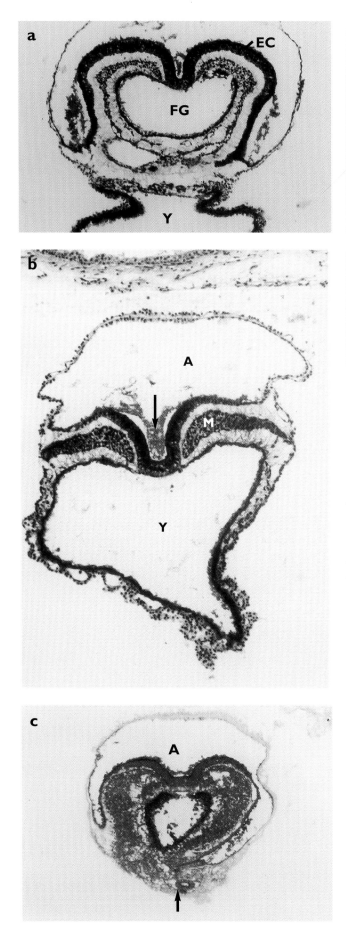

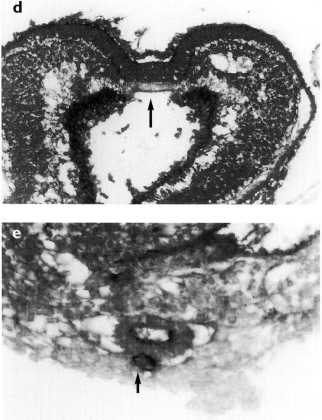

Figure 4.4 Microscopic sections illustrating tissues of an embryo with three pairs of differentiating somites: (a) transverse section of the head with the ectoderm (EC) of a completely open brain primordium, anterior gut (FG) and a paired primordium of the pericardial cavity; (b) transverse section of the middle portion of the embryo: the neural groove (arrow) is completely open; the ventral plate of the neural groove is closely attached to the notochordal plate. Between the ectoderm and the endoderm can be seen the undifferentiated mesodermal plate (M). Within the mesoderm covering the yolk sac (Y) can be seen distinct blood islands; (c) transverse section of the caudal portion of the embryo: in the ceiling of the hindgut can be seen a remnant of the notochordal canal. Within the connecting stalk is the tubule of the allantois with one germ cell (red (arrow)). There is no sharp border between the neuroectoderm and surface ectoderm at this stage; (d) notochordal plate (arrow) at higher magnification; (e) the allantois with germ cell (arrow) at higher magnification. (A – amniotic vesicle)

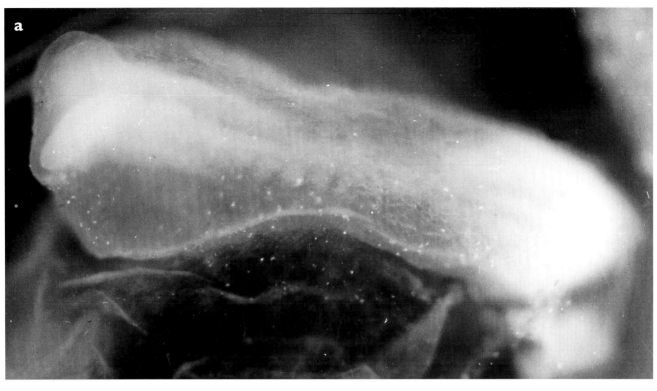

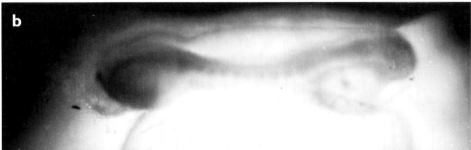

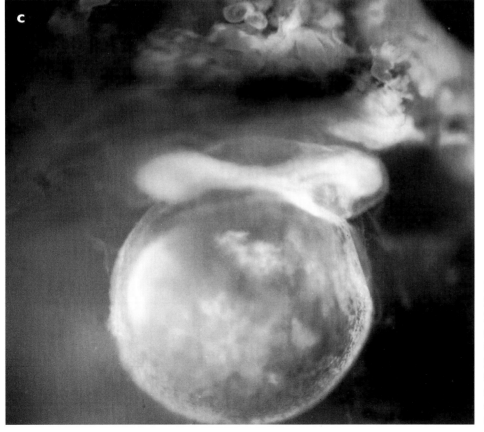

Figure 4.5 (a) Dorsal view of a 23–24-day-old (approximately 2 mm) embryo with nine paired somites: the neural tube is closing at the fifth pair of somites. Open primordia of three brain vesicles are present; (b) lateral view of the same embryo under translucent conditions; (c) lateral view of the same embryo with yolk sac

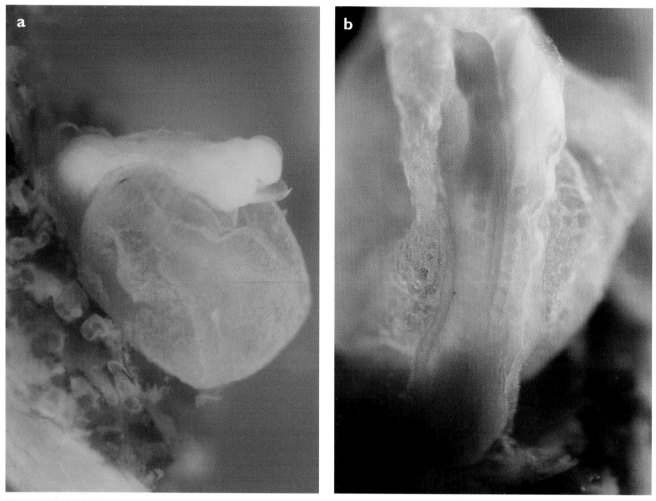

Figure 4.6 (a) A 24–25-day-old (2.5 mm) embryo with 12–13 paired somites, located within the amniotic sac on top of a huge yolk sac, attached to the chorion; (b) the same embryo photographed from the right side: the heart loop is located within the pericardial cavity, adjacent to the yolk sac. This heart loop is already beating

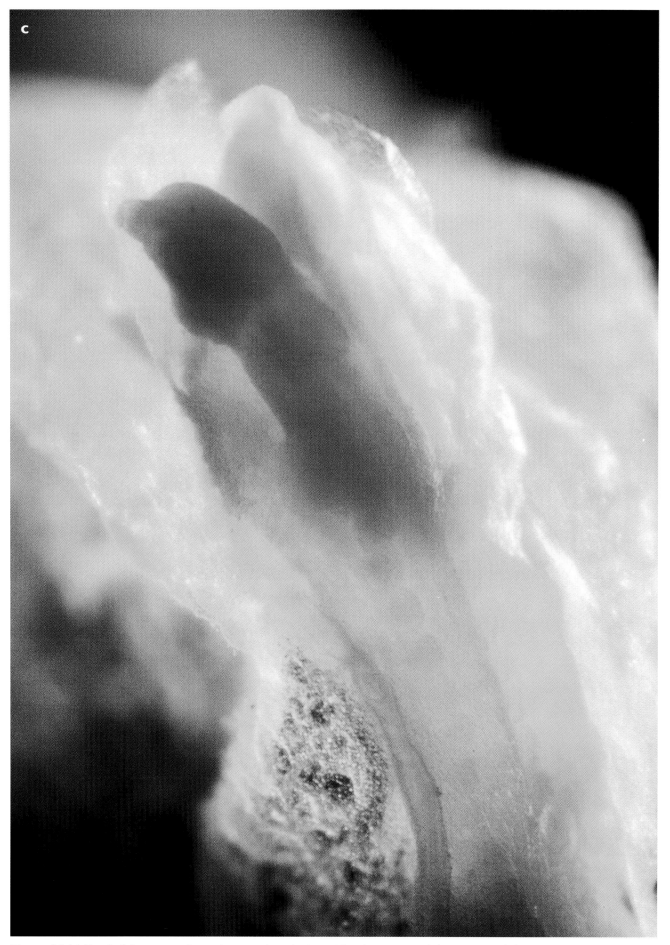

Figure 4.6 (c) Detail of the same embryo: there are three brain vesicles, the prosencephalon, mesencephalon and metencephalon. The prosencephalon is completely open. The most anterior folds on each side of the prosencephalon are the primordia of the optic cups (future retina of the eyes)

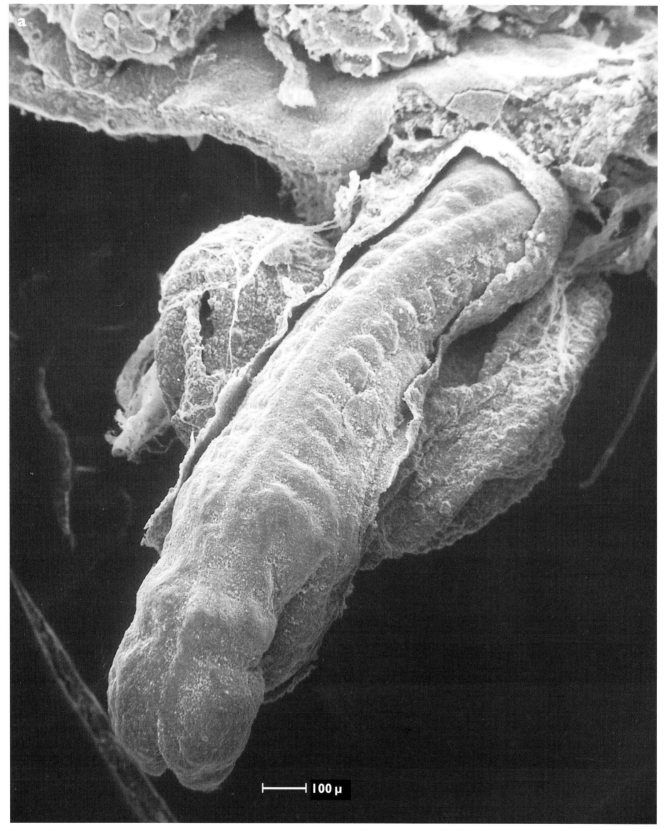

Figure 4.7 Scanning electron micrographs of a 26–27-day-old (2.5 mm) embryo with 14 paired somites, located on the yolk sac: the amniotic sac has been dissected. (a) The three cerebral vesicles are closed (except for anterior and posterior neuropores). Somites are evident on both sides along the closed neural tube; (b) the embryo attached by the connecting stalk to the chorion; (c) lateral view

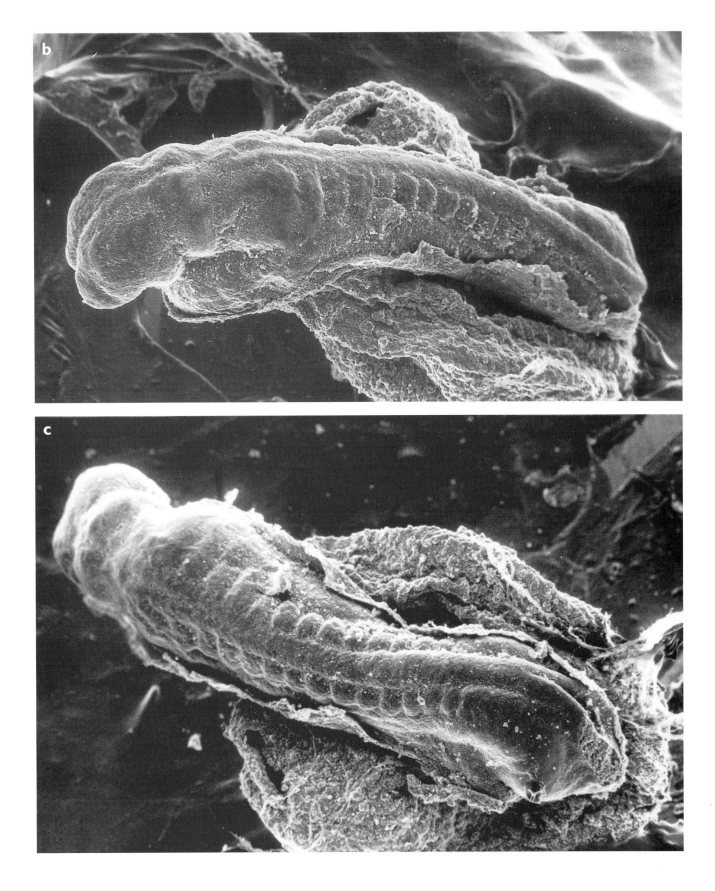

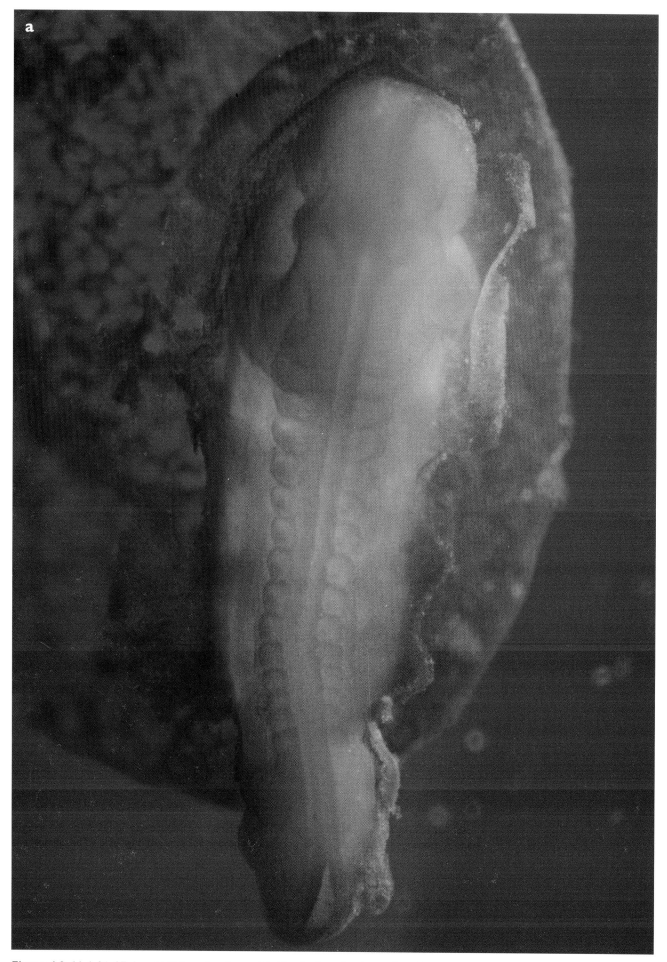

Figure 4.8 (a) A 26–27-day-old (3.0 mm) embryo with 17 paired somites located on the yolk sac
and illuminated by blue light: the anterior neuropore is almost closed, the caudal neuropore is open

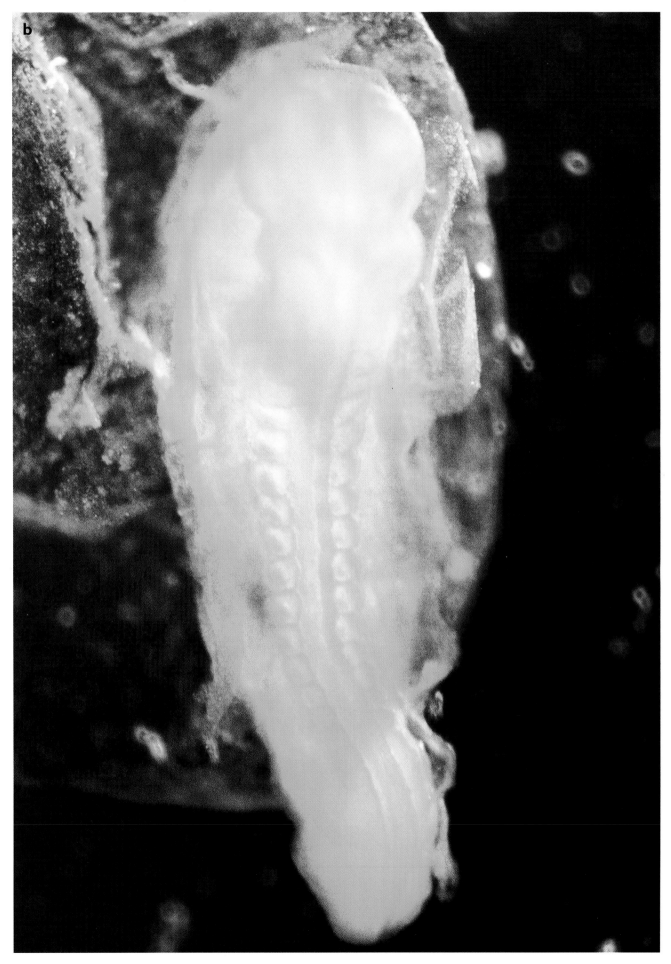

Figure 4.8 (b) The embryo is concave dorsally, related to the separation of the notochord from the closing neural tube

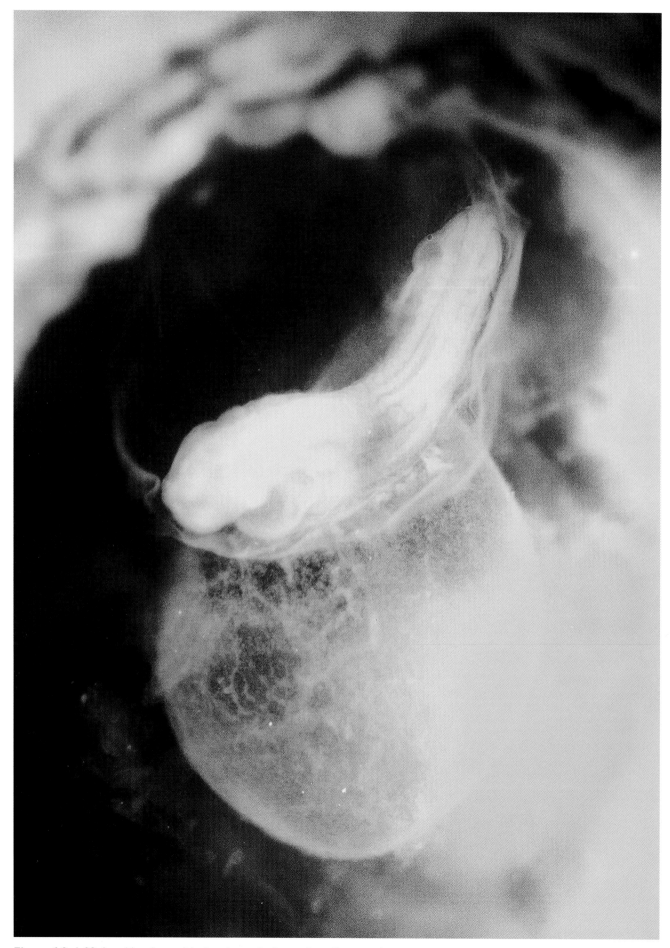

Figure 4.9 A 29-day-old embryo with closed neural tube on the yolk sac: at this stage, in connection
with the positional changes of the notochord, the dorsally concave curvature of the body is very distinct.
The amniotic sac is enlarged by an increasing amount of amniotic fluid

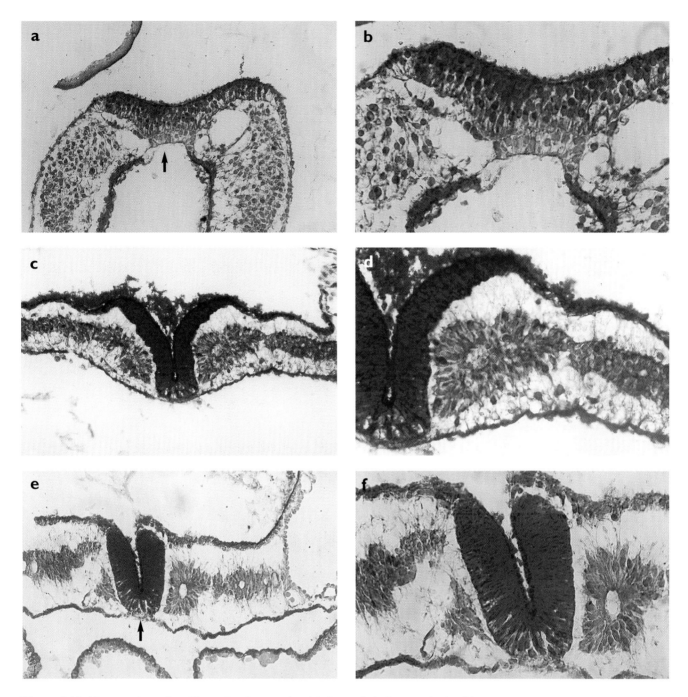

Figure 4.10 Microscopic sections illustrating the notochordal plate and closing neural tube: (a) cross-section of a caudal portion of a pre-somite embryo (19 days). The notochordal plate (arrow) is incorporated in the midline into the ceiling of the yolk sac and is closely attached to the ectoderm. This is the stage of neuroectodermal differentiation; (b) the same as (a) at higher magnification; (c) closing neural tube and differentiation of dorsal mesoderm into somites: between the mesodermal cells and cells of the neuroectoderm and surface ectoderm, long processi of neurodermal cells mediate cell-to-cell interactions; (d) the same as (c) at higher magnification; (e) closing neural tube in an embryo with seven somite pairs: at this stage a distinct border appears between the neuroepithelium (neuroectoderm) of the future neural tube and the surface epithelium. The notochordal plate (arrow) adheres to the ventral plate of the neural groove and, at this stage, inhibits growth of the contracting neuroepithelial cell. This interaction is related to the formation of the medullary ventral plate; (f) the same as (e) at higher magnification

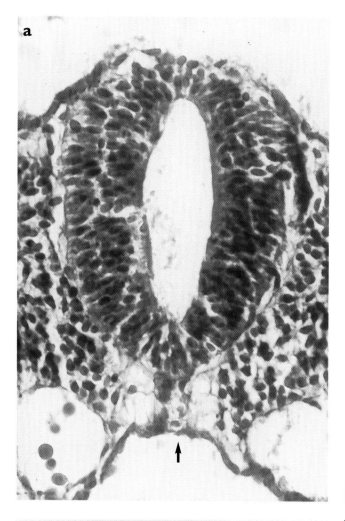

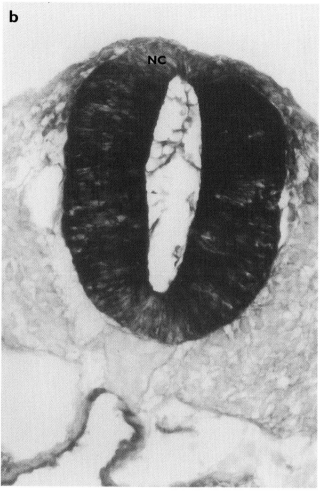

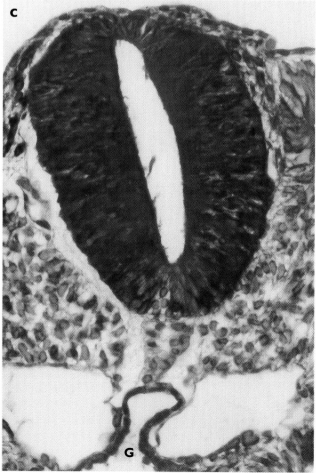

Figure 4.11 Separation of the notochord and proliferation of neural crest (microscopic sections): (a) the notochord (arrow) interposed between the medullary tube and the gut represents the axis of the embryonic body; (b) the notochord acquires a glucosaminoglycan-rich capsule. The medullary tube has a dorsally incomplete external limiting membrane. There are proliferating cells of neural crest (NC); (c) cross-section of the neural tube with proliferating neuroectodermal cells of neural crest: the notochord is detached from the neural tube and gut (G)

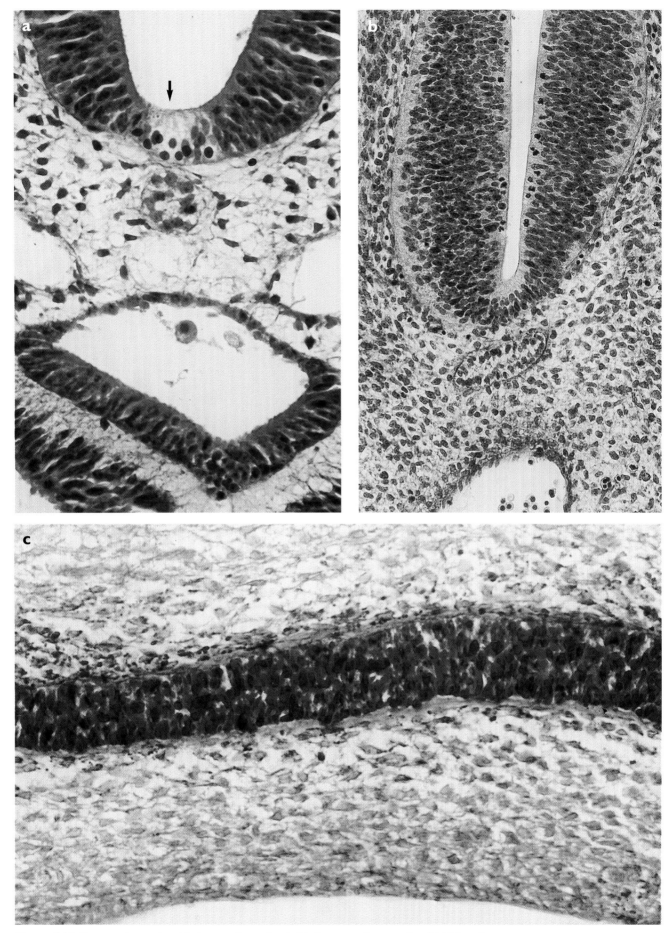

Figure 4.12 Separated notochord (microscopic sections): (a) the separating notochord inhibits adjacent neuroectodermal cells (arrow) of the ventral plate of the medullary tube; (b) the notochord separated from the medullary tube acquires a distinct capsule rich in glucosaminoglycans and becomes the axis of the vertebral column; (c) longitudinal section of the encapsulated notochord: the glycogen, present in notochordal cells, appears red

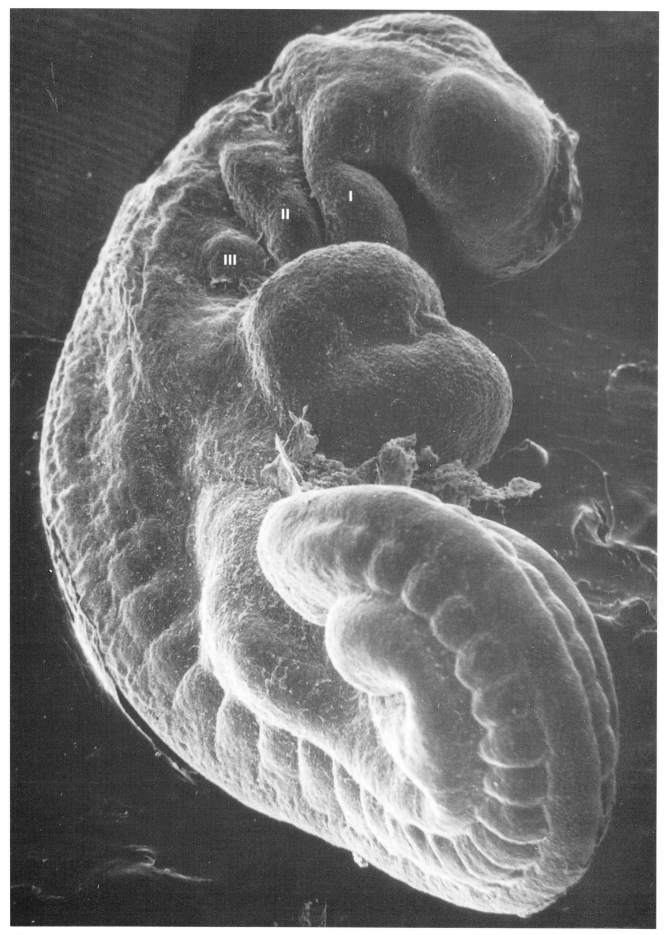

Figure 5.1 Scanning electron micrographs of a 30–32-day-old (4 mm) embryo with 22 paired somites: view from the left side; the yolk sac has been removed. Note three pharyngeal arches (I, II, III); beneath the arches is the bulging aortopulmonary segment of the heart, and anterior to the somites is a very distinct plate of lateral mesoderm

a

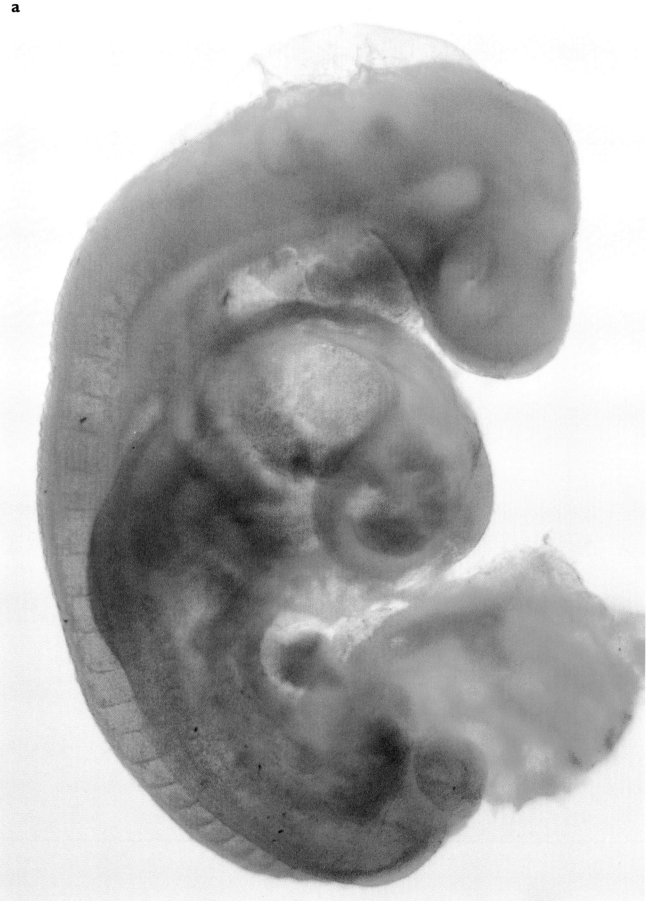

Figure 5.2 (a) C-shaped, 32-day-old (4 mm) embryo with 30 somite pairs showing distinct pharyngeal arches and pouches, heart loop within the pericardial cavity and primordium of the anterior limb bud

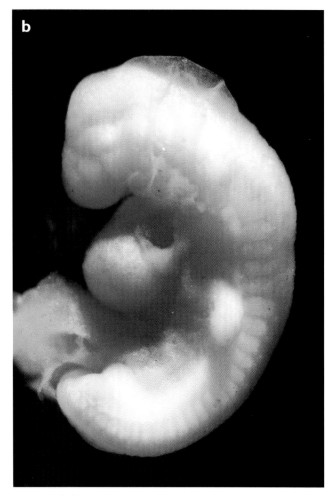

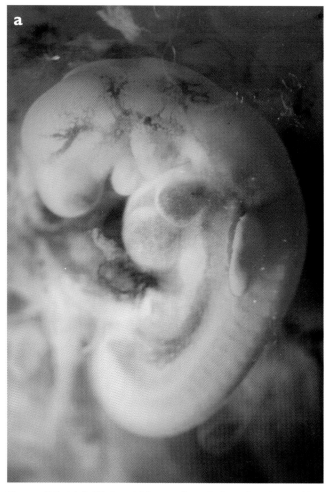

Figure 5.2 (b) The same embryo under different illumination: the anterior limb bud is evident

Figure 5.3 (a) A 35-day-old (approximately 5 mm) embryo with adjacent chorion: the vessels appear black; the anterior limb bud is distinct

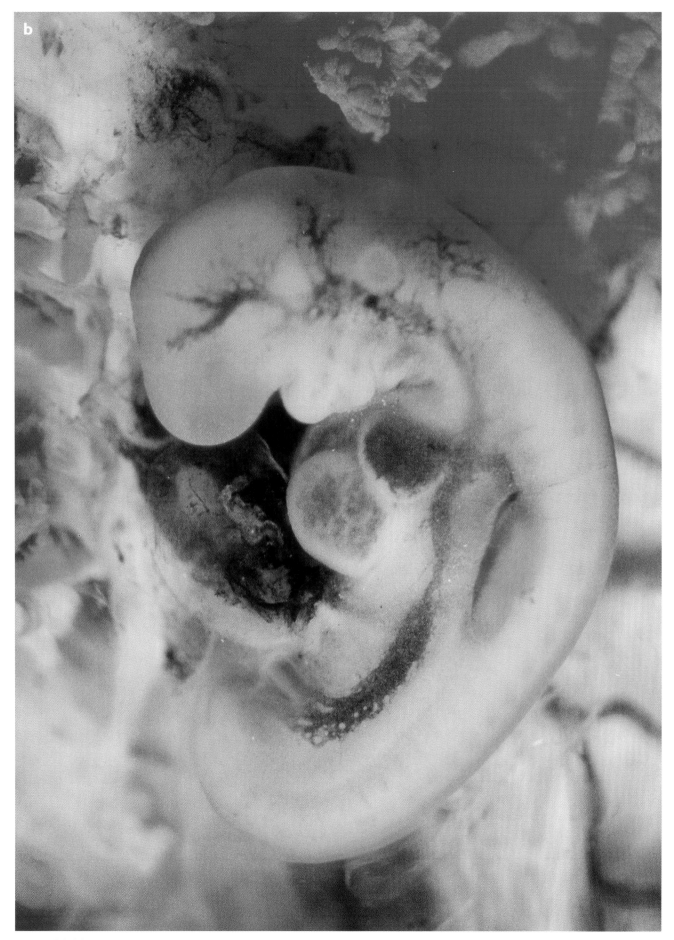

Figure 5.3 (b) The same embryo, demonstrating early embryonic veins entering the heart sinus: the atrial and ventricular segments of the heart loop are separated by the atrioventricular constriction

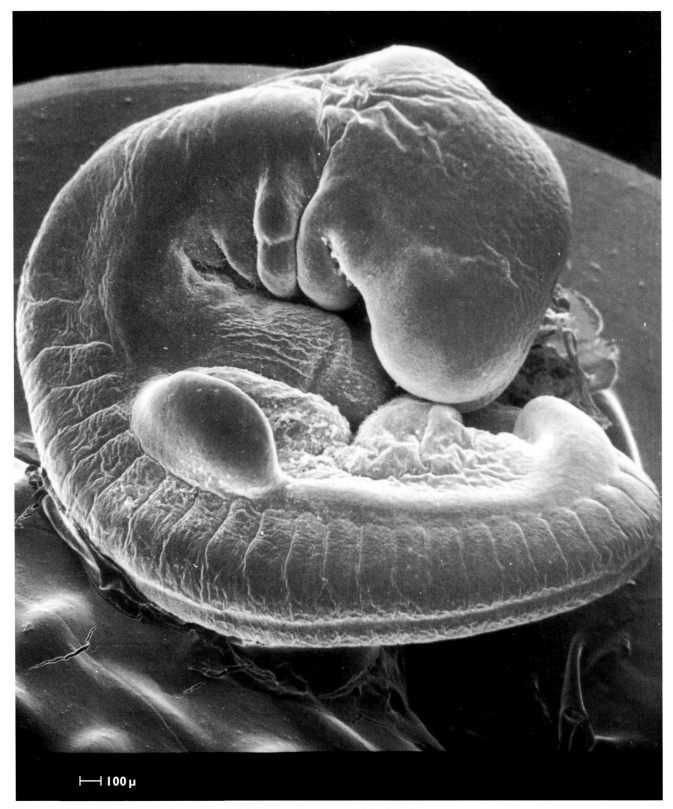

⊢—⊣ 100 μ

Figure 5.4 Scanning electron micrograph of a 34–36-day-old embryo with limb buds

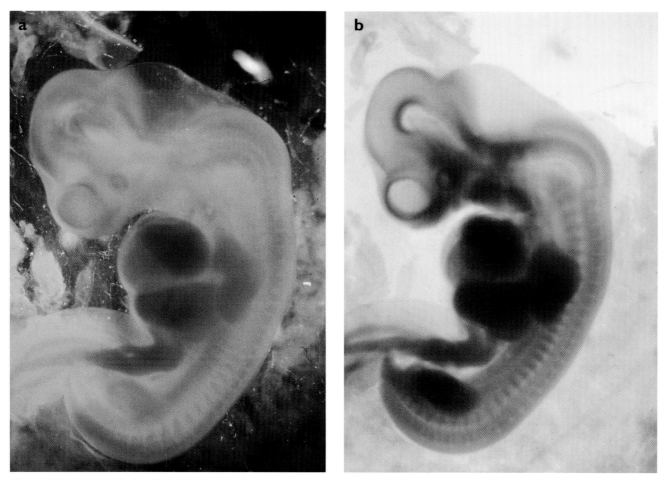

Figure 5.5 (a) A 37–38-day-old (approximately 8 mm) embryo viewed from the left side: ventrally, in the abdominal area, the heart and liver can be seen as well as a distended umbilical vein originating from the fusion of two primitive umbilical veins; (b) translucent view of the same embryo: the embryo exhibits buds of anterior and posterior limbs

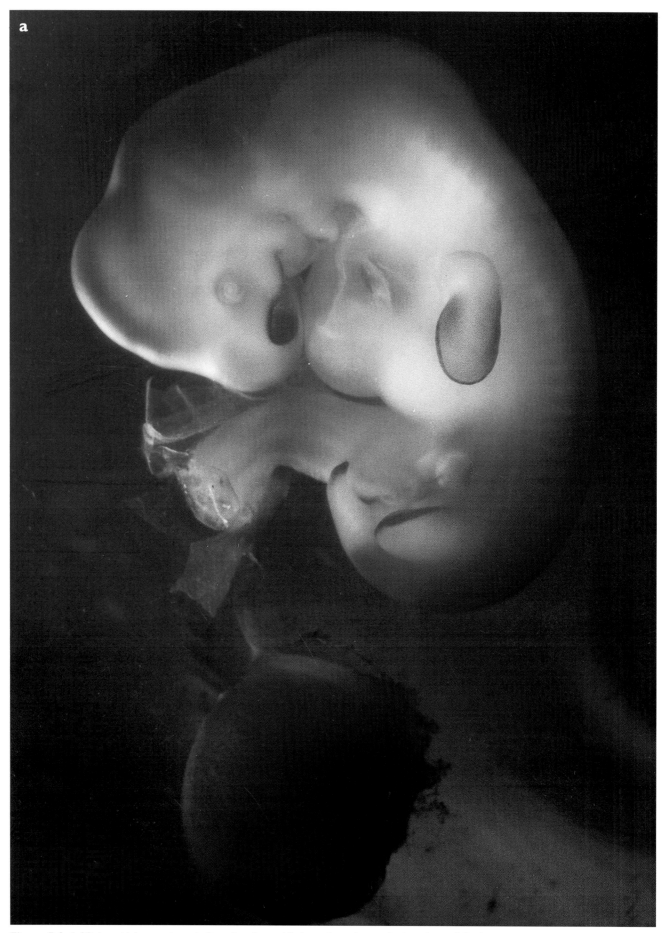

Figure 5.6 A 38-day-old (approximately 9 mm) embryo: (a) the yolk sac is attached to the umbilical cord. The proximal limb has two segments, the distal one a simple limb bud. In the facial area, a distinct olfactory placode can be seen, with an adjacent brain hemisphere. In the occipital area, a relatively large fourth brain ventricle can be distinguished. The body of the embryo ends with a prominent tail

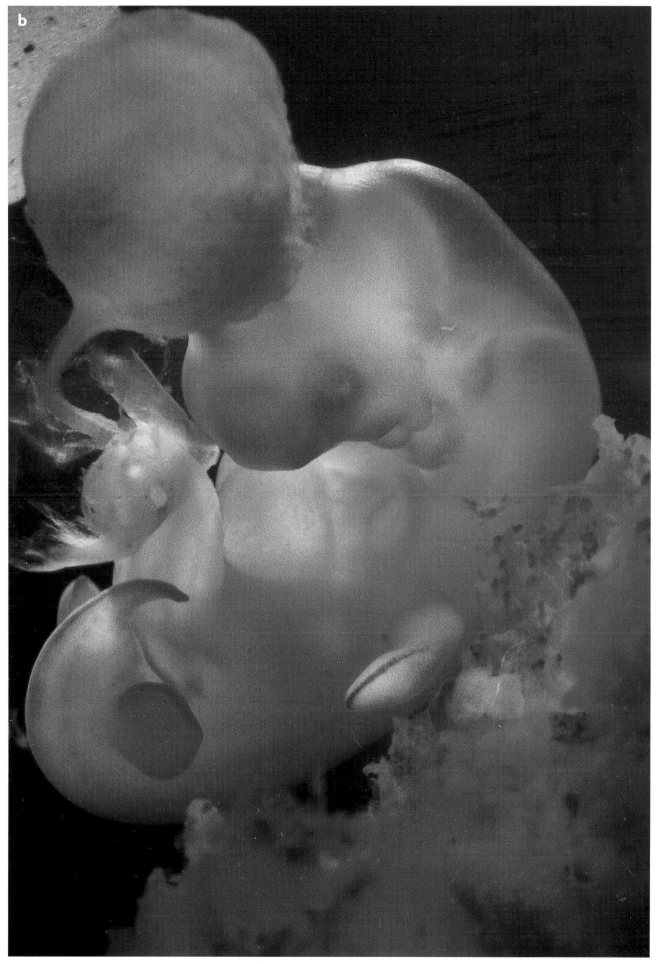

Figure 5.6 (b) The same embryo with yolk sac and chorion

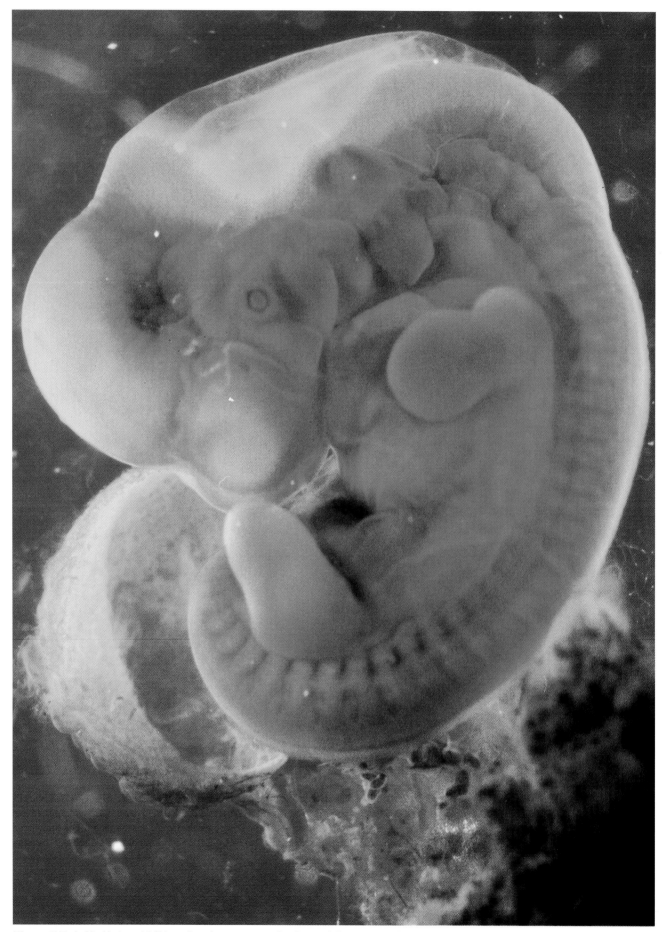

Figure 5.7 A 40–41-day-old (11 mm) embryo: as a result of special illumination, this embryo appears green, which makes the different growth centers and blastemas more distinct. The proximal limb has two distinct segments: the hand plate and the antebrachiobrachial segment. The distal limb has become bisegmented. On the back of the embryo, the double segmentation is related to spinal ganglia and sclerotomes, contributing vertebral primordia

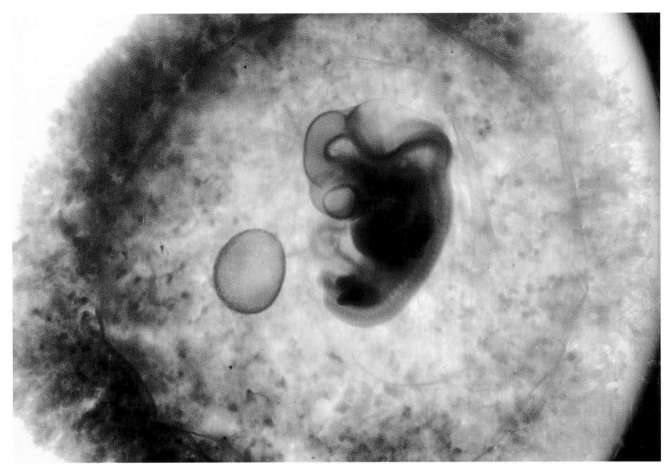

Figure 5.8 Translucent view of a 42–43-day-old (12 mm) embryo with chorion and yolk sac

a

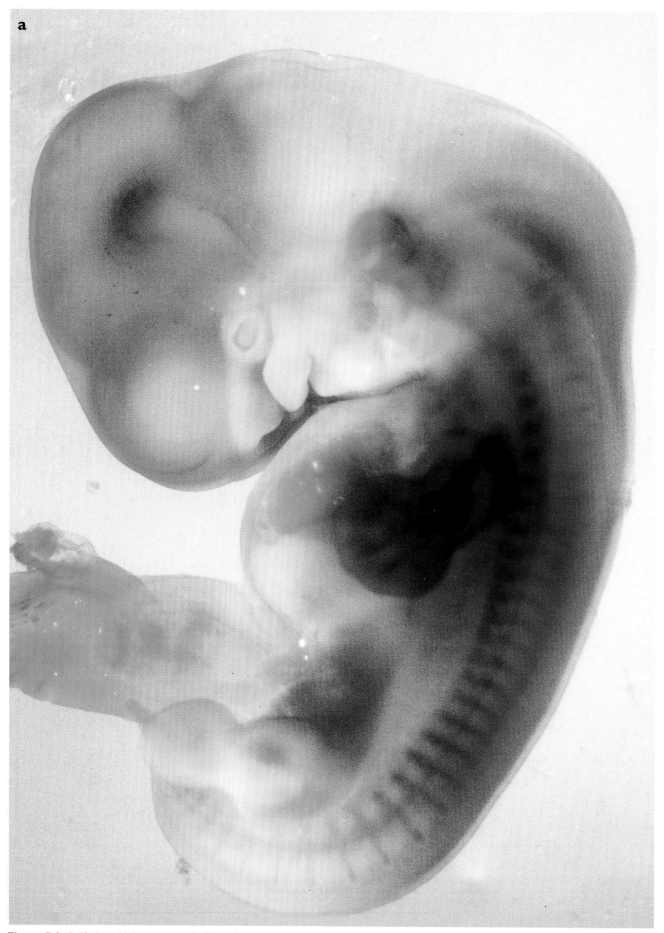

Figure 5.9 A 43-day-old (approximately 13 mm) embryo: (a) fluorescent illumination makes the structures of the face very distinct. Anterior and posterior limbs are bisegmented

b

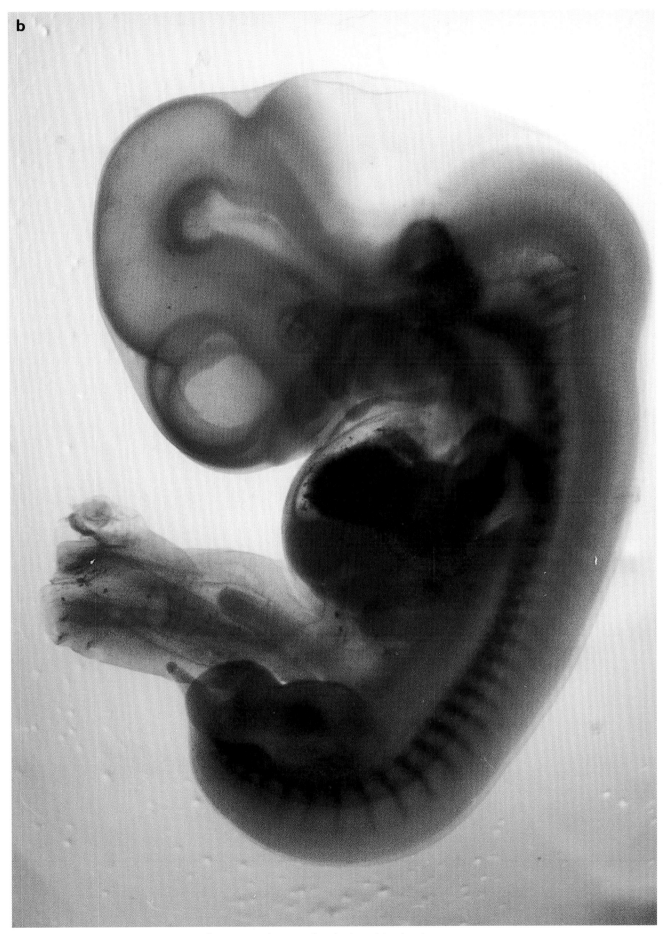

(b) The same embryo under translucent illumination: the secondary brain vesicles, i.e. the
telencephalon with hemispheres, the diencephalon, the mesencephalon, the metencephalon and the
myelencephalon are evident. The fourth cerebral ventricle is prominent

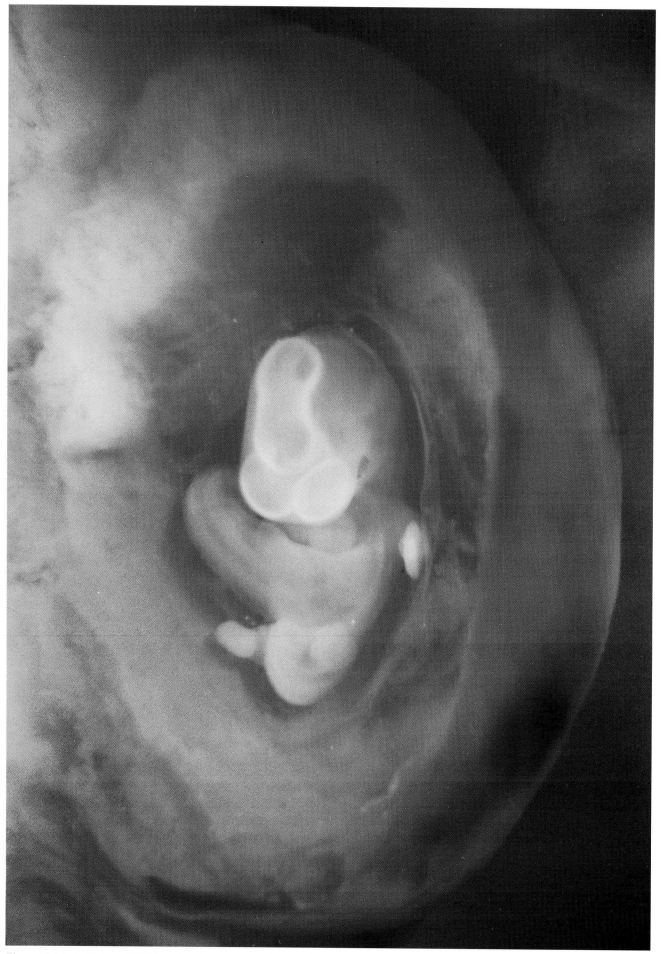

Figure 5.10 A 43-day-old (12.5 mm) embryo implanted within the uterus: the chorion (gestational sac) is covered by decidua and the embryo, located within the amniotic sac, is attached to the villous chorion by a thick umbilical cord

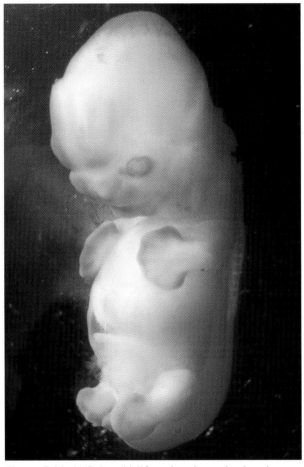

Figure 5.11 A 45-day-old (13 mm) embryo: the dorsal segmentation becomes indistinct. Early tubercles of fingers are present

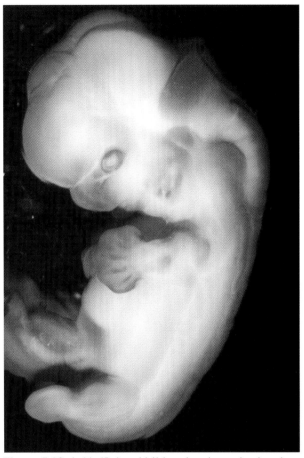

Figure 5.12 A 44–45-day-old (14 mm) embryo: the dorsal segmentation has faded, and the pharyngeal arches have disappeared. The pinna is formed around the external auditory meatus. The growth centers of the face are indistinct. Finger tubercles, related to cartilaginous finger rays (blue) can be seen on the hand plates

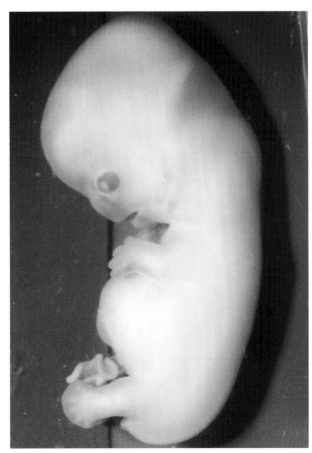

Figure 5.13 A 47–48-day-old (17 mm) embryo with a distinct face and eyes without eyelids. Finger tubercles are present while on the foot plates only toe rays can be seen

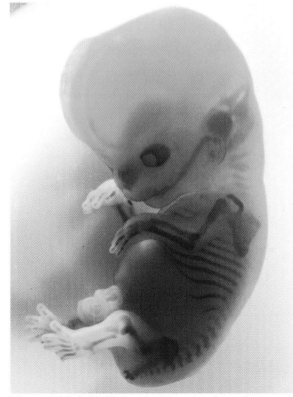

Figure 5.14 A 56–57-day-old (28 mm) embryo photographed under translucent conditions: fingers and toes are differentiated; cerebral hemispheres are distinct. The eyes are dark as a result of the dark brown pigment, melanin, present within the retina

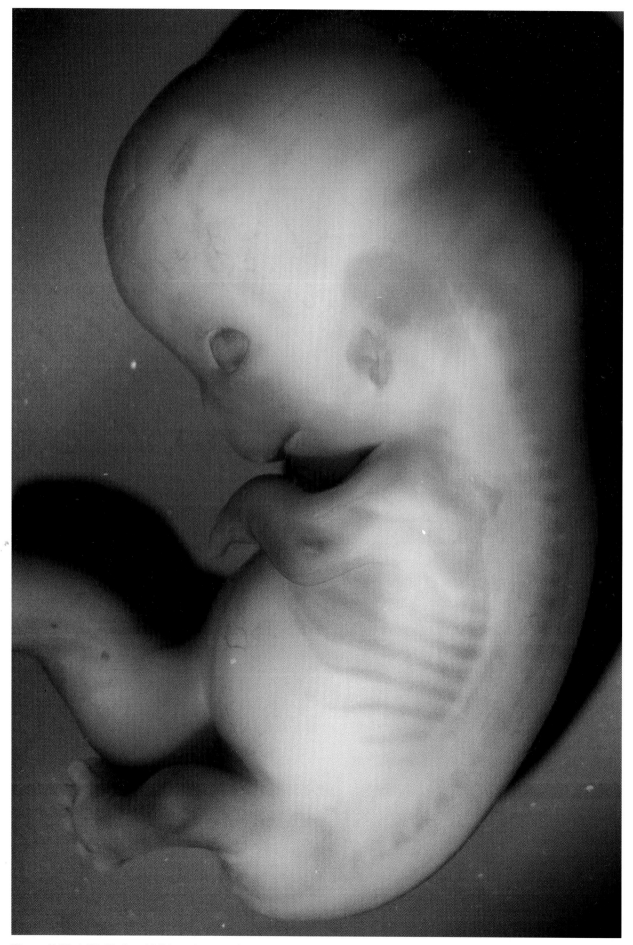

Figure 5.15 A 51–52-day-old (22 mm) embryo: the cartilages are blue. The umbilical cord is thick as the gut loops evaginate into its proximal portion. This condition represents the physiological umbilical hernia. Fingers and toes are evident

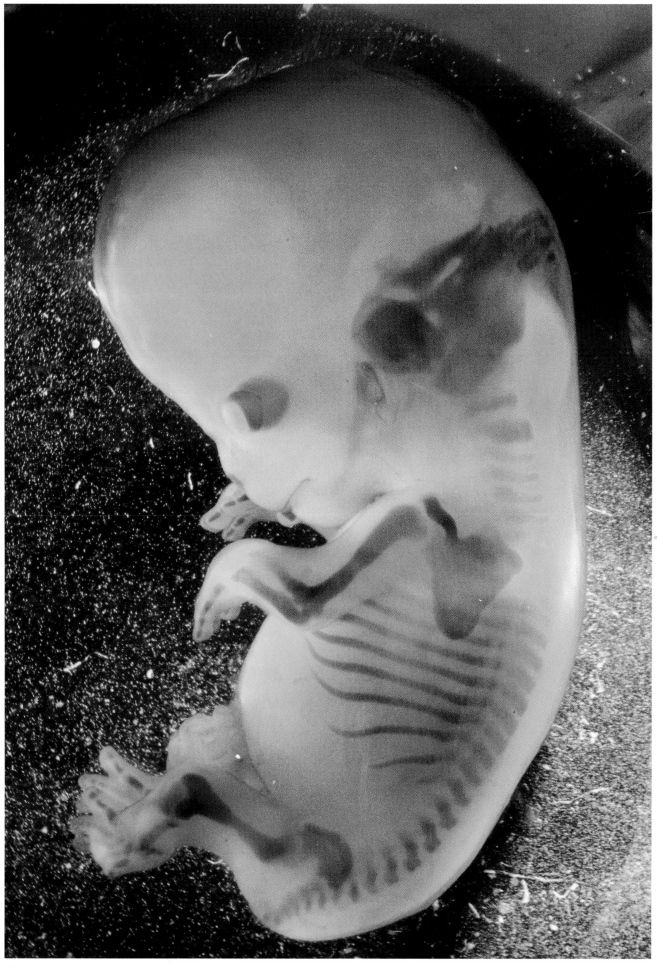

Figure 5.16 A 57-day-old (27 mm) embryo with visualized chondroskeleton: 'models' of bones formed by cartilages

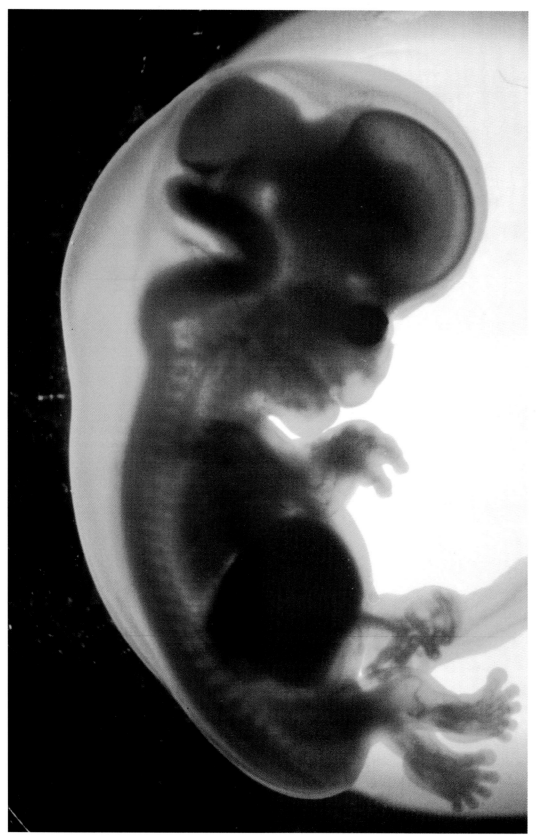

Figure 5.17 Early fetus (38 mm) from the beginning of the 11th gestational week, affected by nuchal translucency: nuchal translucency is an important unspecific marker of early fetal maldevelopment and represents the accumulation of fluid, which originates as the cerebrospinal liquor of the fourth cerebral ventricle. The fluid diffuses dorsally into the subcutaneous connective tissue and accumulates between the cutaneous connective tissue and the superficial fascia of the body, if the venous drainage of this space is insufficient. This happens when the blood circulation is failing, such as in fetuses with congenital heart defects or with chronic hypoxia, and appears in many fetuses affected by various chromosomal aneuploidies, including Down's syndrome. Nuchal translucency is a 'window phenomenon' of embryonic and early fetal maldevelopment seen between gestational weeks 9 and 18, and is related to the separation of the intracranial and extracranial space. As the neural arches of the vertebrae become closed and the squama of the occipital bone develops, the liquor formed by the stria terminalis and the choroid plexus of the fourth cerebral ventricle can no longer pass into the subcutaneous space

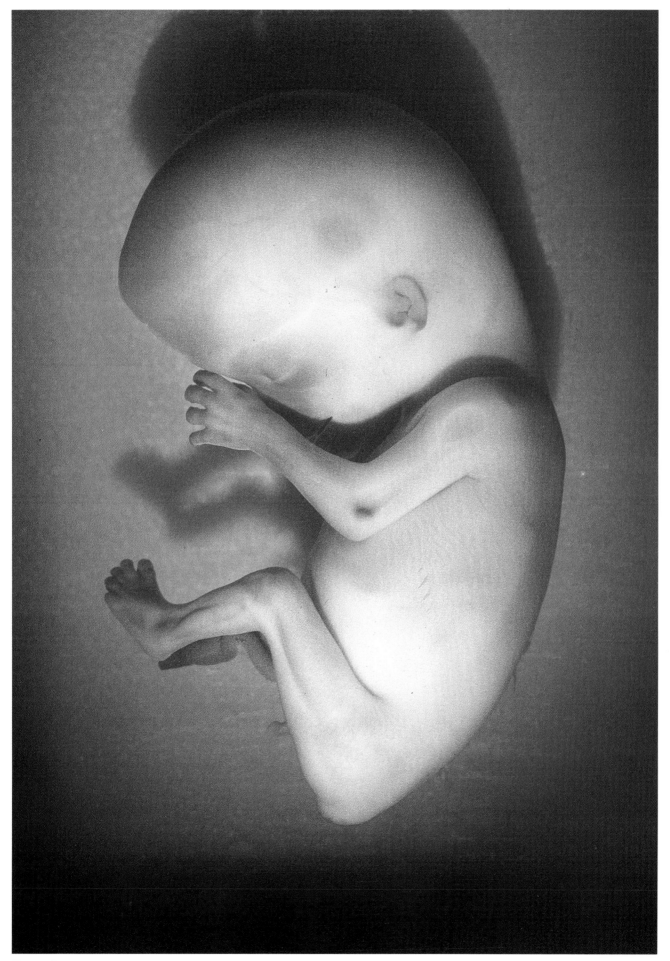

Figure 6.1 The early fetus appears fully human: the eyes are closed, and the crown–rump length is approximately 45 mm, 13th gestational week

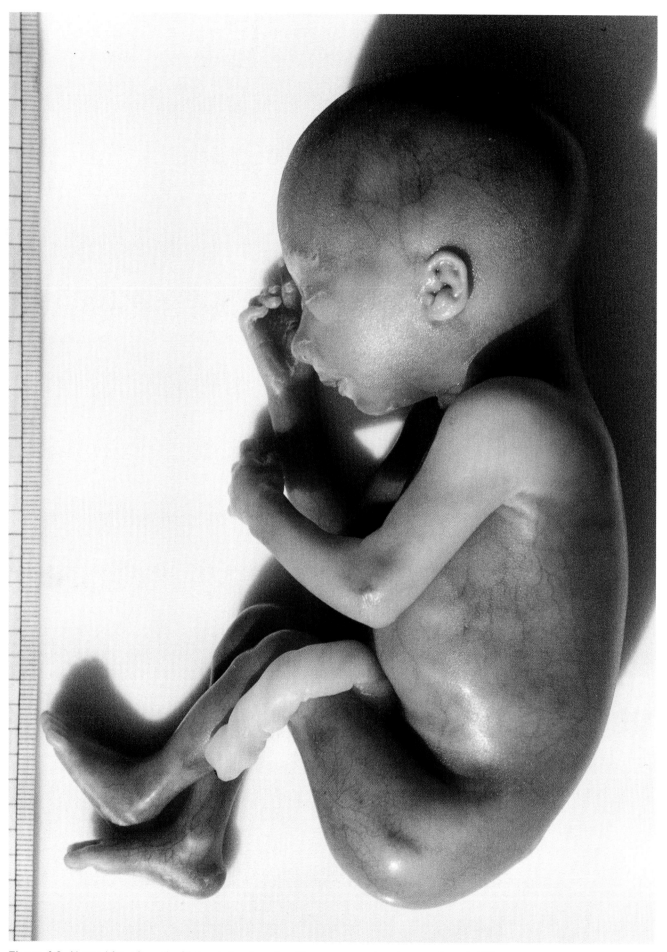

Figure 6.2 Aborted fetus from the 21st gestational week, with crown–rump length approximately 180mm, total body weight 220g: such a fetus is unable to survive. The eyelids are fused. The morphology of the fetus is similar to that of the newborn

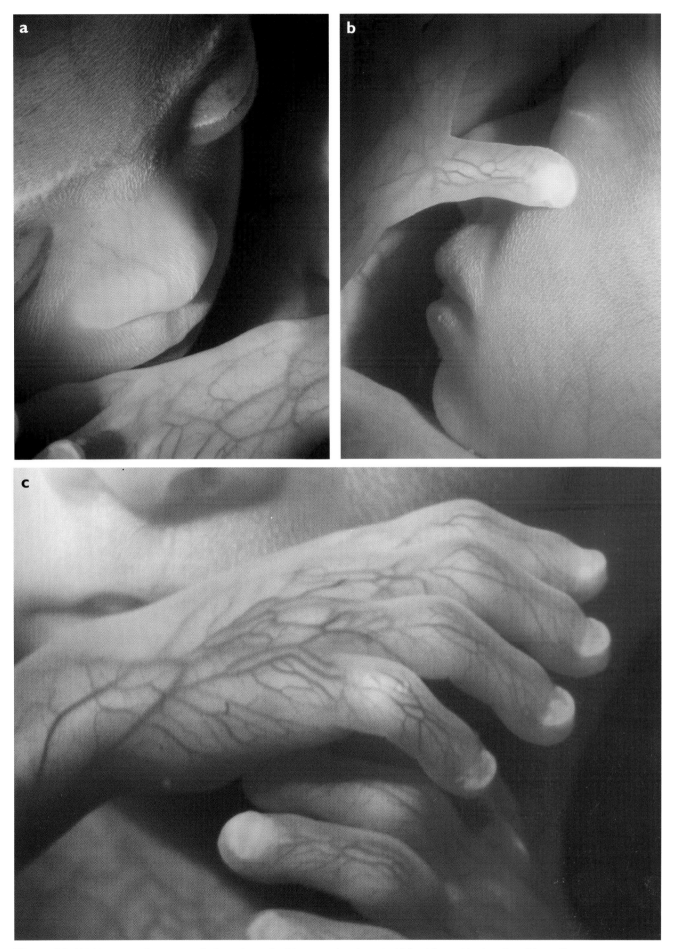

Figure 6.3 Within-uterus fetoscopy of a fetus from the 21st gestational week: (a) fetal face with closed eyelids, well-formed nose and upper lip; the hands show distinct veins; (b) fused eyelids and very short eyelashes; (c) the hands show a pattern of veins, and fingers with nails

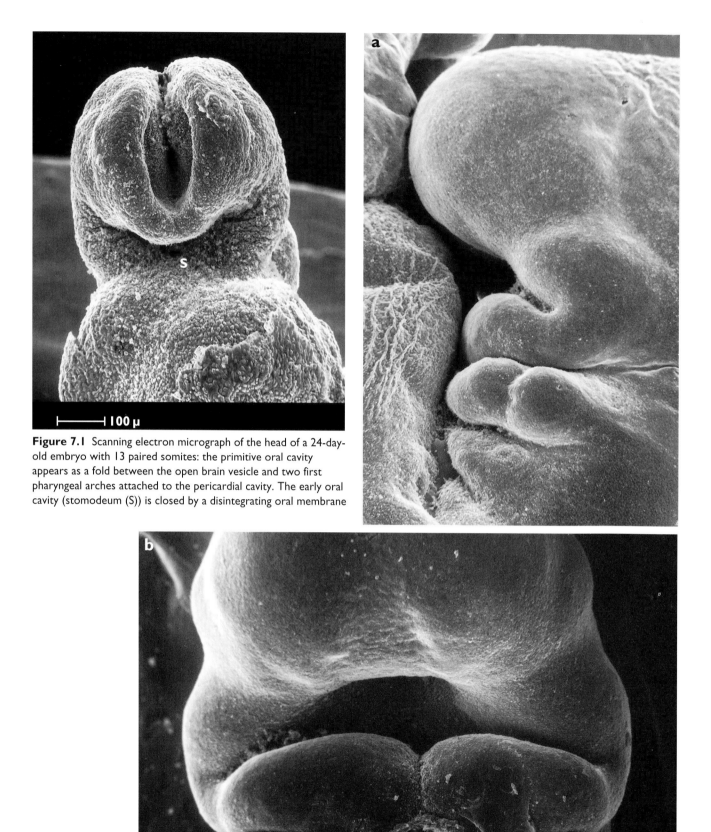

Figure 7.1 Scanning electron micrograph of the head of a 24-day-old embryo with 13 paired somites: the primitive oral cavity appears as a fold between the open brain vesicle and two first pharyngeal arches attached to the pericardial cavity. The early oral cavity (stomodeum (S)) is closed by a disintegrating oral membrane

Figure 7.2 Scanning electron micrograph of the head of a 30-day-old embryo: the primitive mouth is delineated by the closed prosencephalic vesicle with optic cups and by the first pharyngeal arches. The maxillary primordium can be seen on the first pharyngeal arches. (a) Lateral view; (b) frontal view

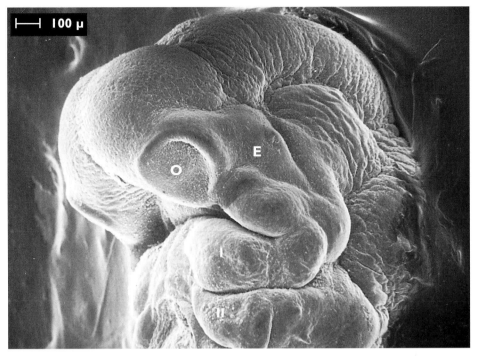

Figure 7.3 Scanning electron micrograph of the head of a 36–37-day-old embryo: the horseshoe-shaped early olfactory groove (O) is connected to the eye (E) by oculonasal mesenchyme. The first pharyngeal arches (I) fuse into a single mandibular arch (second pharyngeal arch – II)

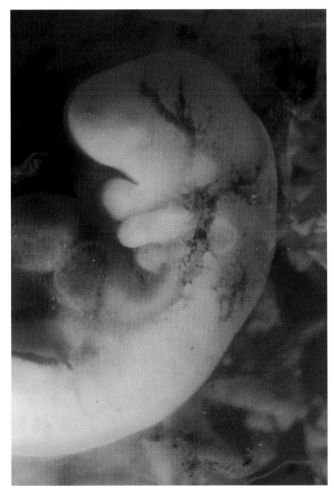

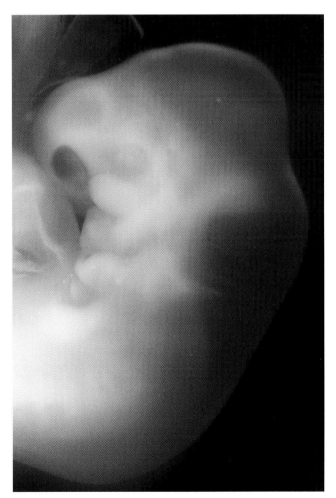

Figure 7.4 Profile of a 35-day-old (5 mm) embryo: the early veins appear black. The indistinct olfactory placode is located rostrally on the most prominent prosencephalic portion of the head. Underneath is the fold of the primitive oral cavity, delineated by the first pharyngeal arches. The second, third and fourth pharyngeal arches are present in the area of the neck

Figure 7.5 Profile of a 38-day-old (9 mm) embryo: the former olfactory placode changes into a distinct nasal pit (red) inducing, laterally, proliferation of the oculonasal mesenchyme and, medially, proliferation of the adjacent neuroepithelium of the prosencephalon into the brain hemisphere. In addition, maxillary centers appear on the mandibular arch

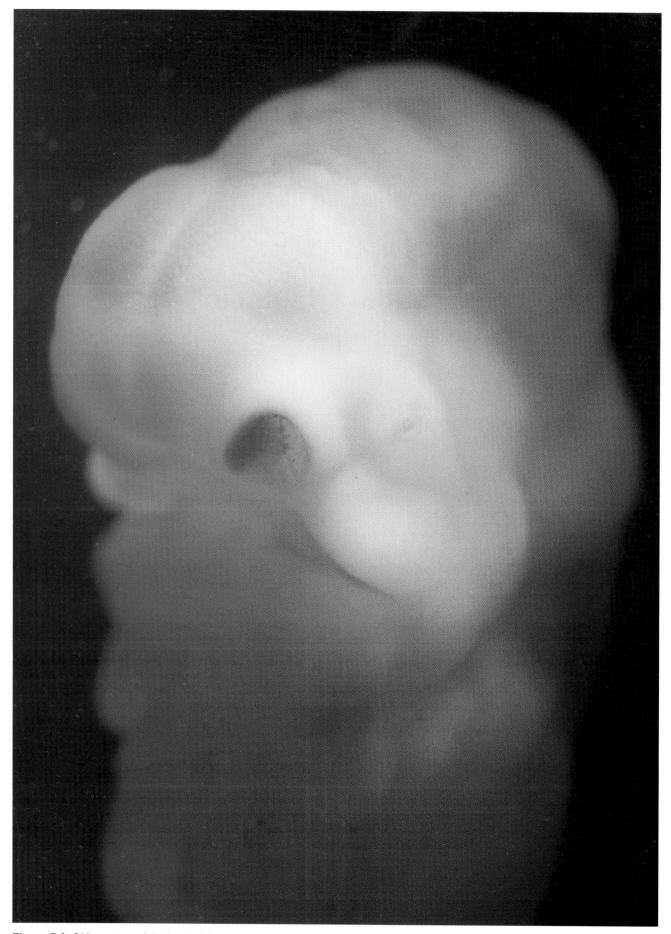

Figure 7.6 Oblique view of the head of the embryo shown in Figure 7.5, demonstrating the nasal pit and the segments of the upper lip: the nasal groove is delineated by the nasal portion of the oculonasal mesenchyme. The lens vesicle of the eye is just closing. The distinct maxillary primordium is separated from the nasal mesenchyme by a deep nasolacrimal furrow. The cerebral hemisphere bulges close to the midline

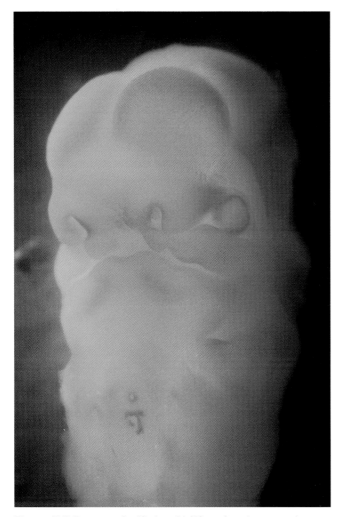

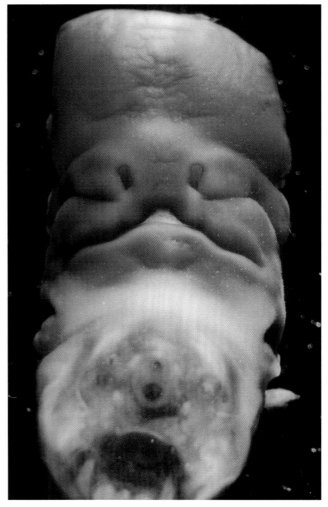

Figure 7.7 Portrait of a 42-day-old (12 mm) embryo: nasal placodes have transformed into nasal pits; each pit is delineated by a nasal ridge. On each ridge, premaxillary, medial nasal and lateral nasal portions are evident. Cerebral hemispheres are bulging in the frontal area of the head. The maxillary primordium and the lateral portion of the nasal ridge are separated by a deep nasolacrimal furrow. The premaxillary portion of the nasal ridge and the maxillary primordium are separated by a deep furrow. The lower lip and jaw are derivatives of the mandibular arch

Figure 7.8 Face of 44-day-old (14 mm) embryo: fusion of the premaxillary portion of the nasal ridge and the maxillary primordium is evident as the embryonic connective tissue penetrates through the junction. A distinct midline field of the dorsum of the nose has formed, related to the nasal capsule and nasal septum. The interocular depression separates the nasal and frontal areas of the face. The nasolacrimal furrows are still very deep

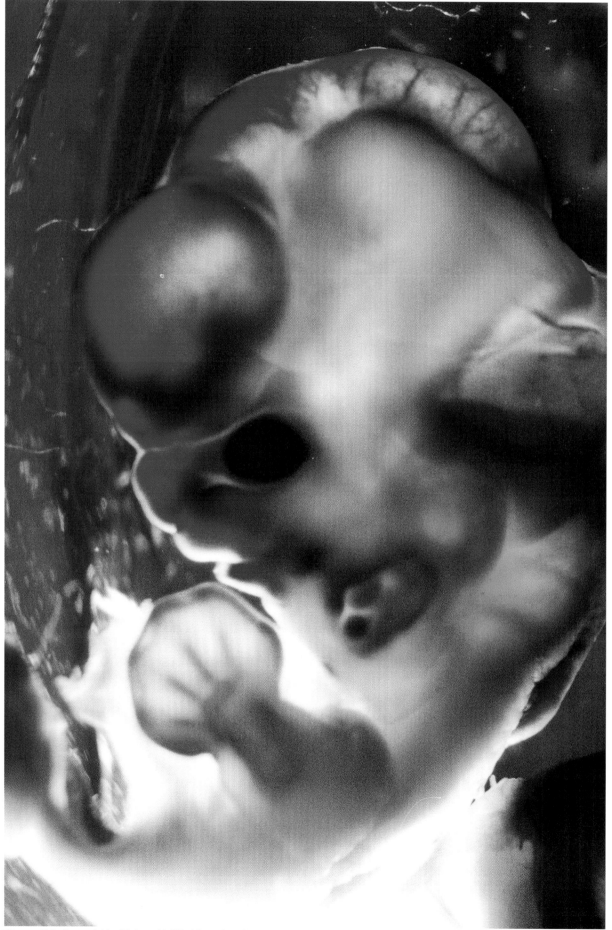

Figure 7.9 Face of 46–47-day-old (18–19 mm) embryo: the brain hemispheres, the mesencephalon with vessels, the eye, nose, mouth and the external ear with adjacent otic capsule are depicted. The hand exhibits early digital tubercles and cartilaginous finger rays

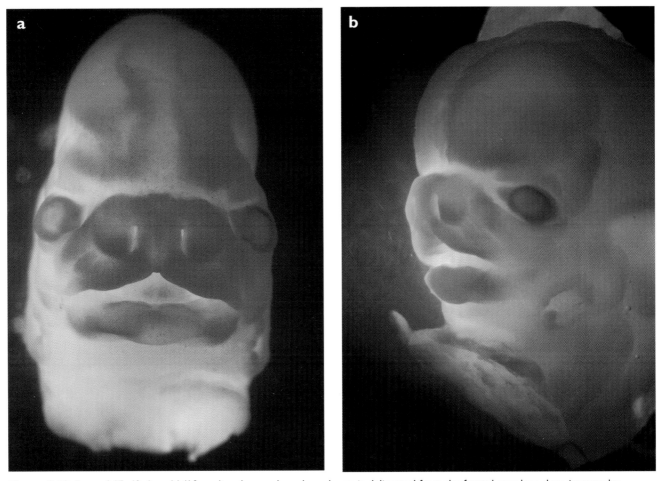

Figure 7.10 Face of 47–49-day-old (18 mm) embryo: a broad nasal area is delineated from the frontal area by a deep interocular depression. The naris is delineated by the lateral portion of the nasal ridge, superiorly near the eye corner, and a stream of zygomatic mesenchyme fills the nasolacrimal furrow, the bottom of which is the nasolacrimal canal. In the midline, there is a distinct primordium of the nose tip, related to the formation of the sagittal nasal septum. Mesenchyme of this septum brings both medial and premaxillary portions of the nasal ridges together. In the midline of the primary lip, there is still a distinct incisure. The frenulum and philtrum of the upper lip are formed by additional midline mesenchymal proliferation, as the midline incisure of the primary lip disappears. (a) Frontal view; (b) oblique view. The pinna is present

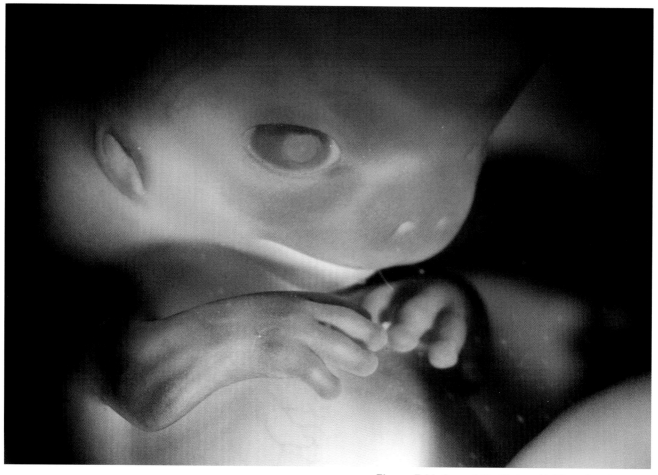

Figure 7.11 Face of 52–53-day-old (23 mm) embryo: the nose is broad and flat. The primary upper lip is completely closed, as the midline incisure has been filled with mesenchyme. On each side, close to the radix of nose, there is a prominent vein, medial from the inner corner of the eye fissure. Primordia of the eyelids are distinct. The pinna delineates the opening of the external auditory meatus

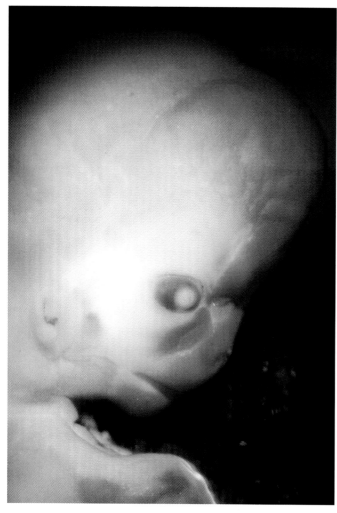

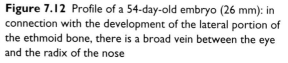

Figure 7.12 Profile of a 54-day-old embryo (26 mm): in connection with the development of the lateral portion of the ethmoid bone, there is a broad vein between the eye and the radix of the nose

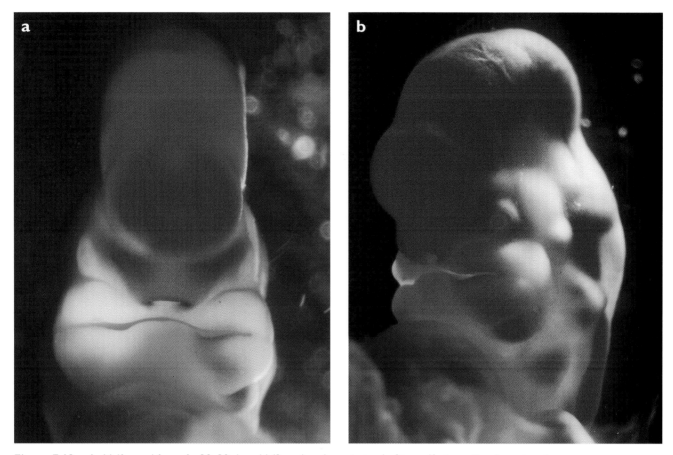

Figure 7.13 a, b Malformed face of a 38–39-day-old (8 mm) embryo: instead of two olfactory pits adjacent to the stomodeum, there is a single pit located in the midline of the upper lip. The upper jaw is contributed by just two maxillary primordia fused in the midline (there is no premaxilla). The circular nasal ridge of the single nasal pit is formed by oculonasal mesenchyme from both sides. The single olfactory placode induces formation of a single midline cerebral vesicle (instead of two hemispheres). This condition is known as holoprosencephaly. The malformed nose with a single nostril is known as ethmocephaly. Premaxillary agenesis, cebocephaly and holoprosencephaly represent a developmental sequence related to a chromosomal aneuploidy, usually trisomy 13. Holoprosencephaly is readily detectable using ultrasound in late embryos at 10–11 gestational weeks (30–35 mm). Over 90% of embryos and fetuses affected by trisomy 13 can be detected in this way

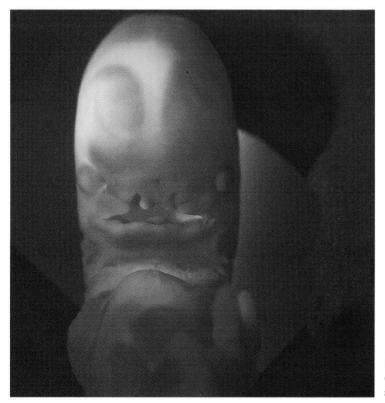

Figure 7.14 Bilateral cleft lip present in a 13-mm embryo: the premaxillary portions of the nasal ridges and the maxillary primordia are separated

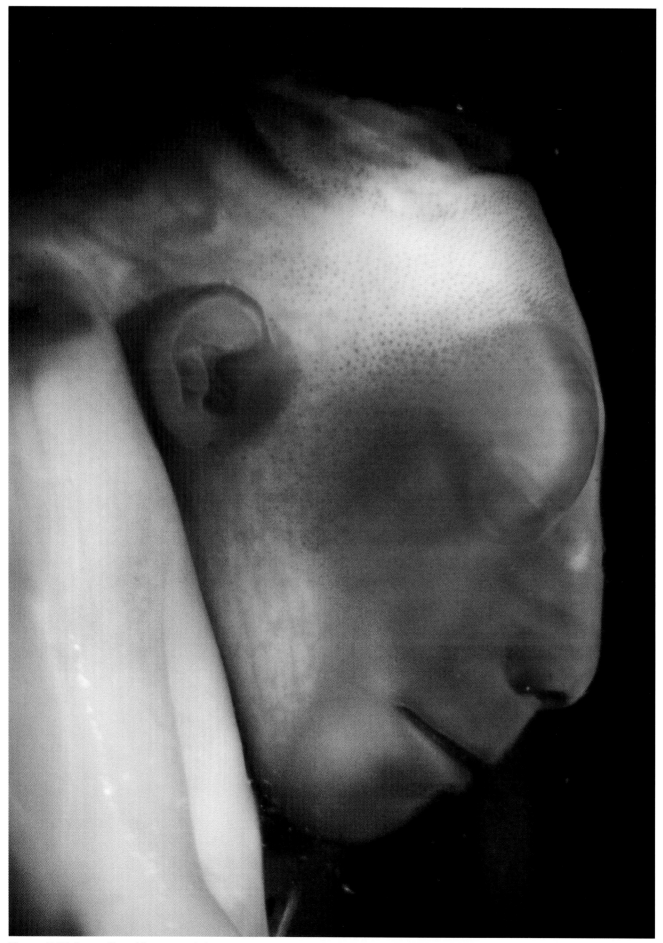

Figure 7.15 Fetus affected by anencephaly, 16th gestational week: anencephaly is incompatible with survival, and represents one of the conditions readily detectable using early ultrasound visualization. In anencephalics, the brain is replaced by a mixture of degenerating brain tissue and irregular vessels

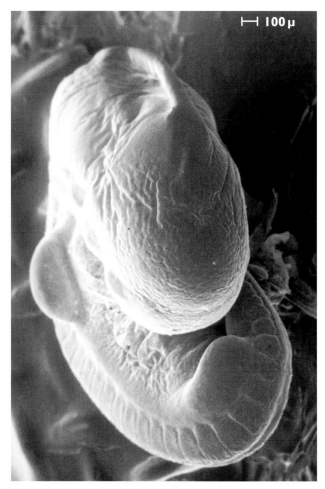

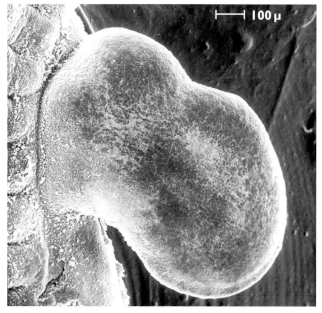

Figure 8.2 Bisegmented right anterior limb with adjacent somites, 8-mm embryo (scanning electron microscopy)

Figure 8.1 Limb buds located on the non-segmented lateral mesodermal plate, 6-mm embryo (scanning electron microscopy)

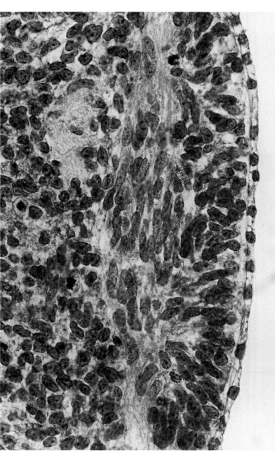

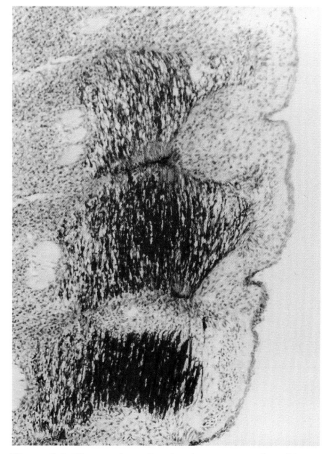

Figure 8.3 Microscopic section of a dermatomyotome: muscle cells (myoblasts) form a bundle of parallel-oriented spindle-shaped cells

Figure 8.4 Microscopic section showing segments of myoblasts (glycogen within myoblasts is stained red)

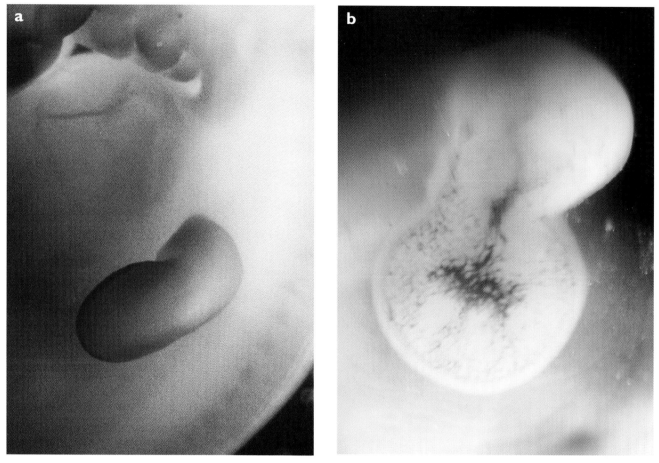

Figure 8.5 The bisegmented limb bud of a 38-day-old embryo: (a) the ectodermal apical
ridge appears red; (b) vasculogenesis

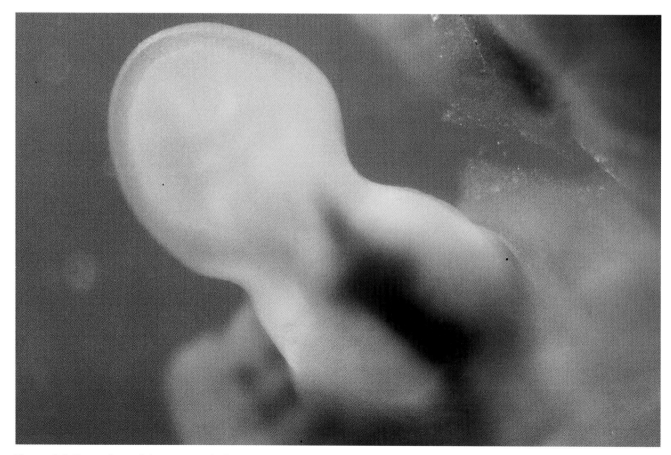

Figure 8.6 Primordium of the posterior limb consisting of a foot plate and a proximal segment:
cartilages of the chondroskeleton (dark blue) appear in the proximo–distal sequence

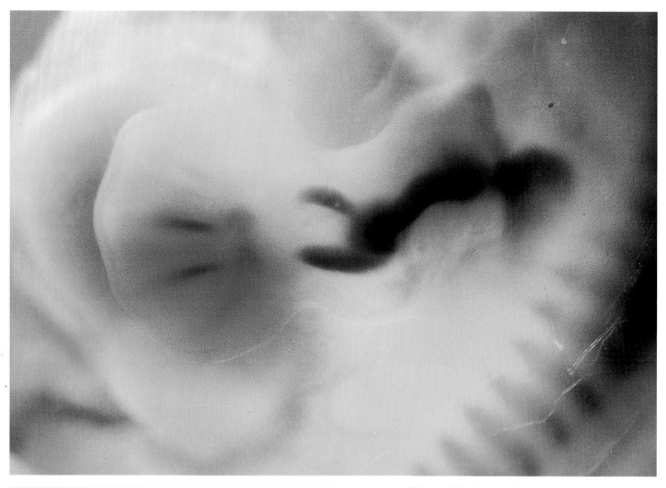

Figure 8.7 Anterior limb showing cartilaginous digital rays and regressing apical cup in a 43-day-old (14 mm) embryo: the center affecting organization of digital rays is located lateral to the little finger

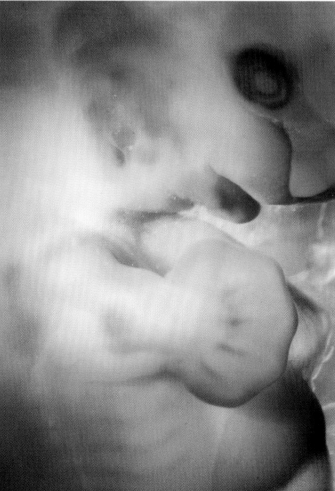

Figure 8.8 46-day-old (17–18 mm) embryo with early digital tubercles and cartilaginous finger rays

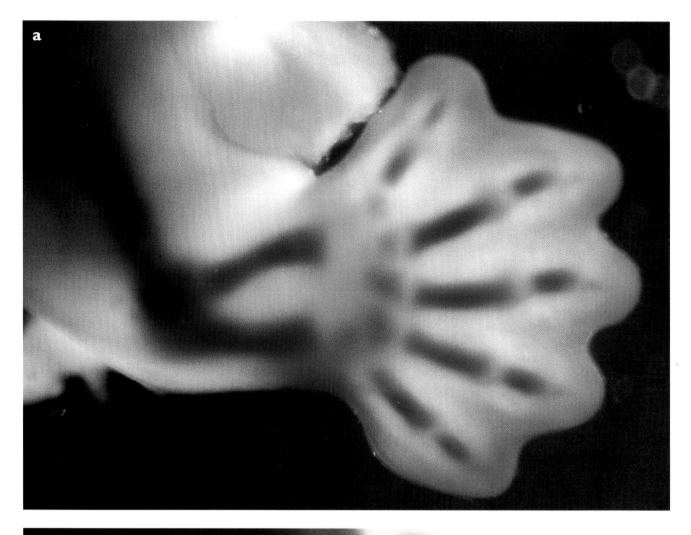

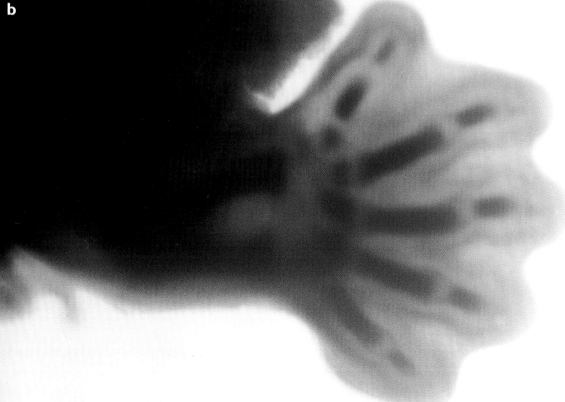

Figure 8.9 (a) Cartilaginous skeleton of the forearm and hand showing primordia of bones and joints; (b) translucent view of the same hand: between digits can be seen distinct lines and fields of apoptosis; most of the original mesenchyme of the limb buds perishes by apoptosis

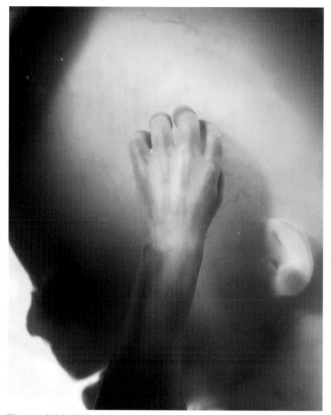

Figure 8.10 Fully differentiated fingers and cartilaginous skeleton in an early fetus from the 12th gestational week

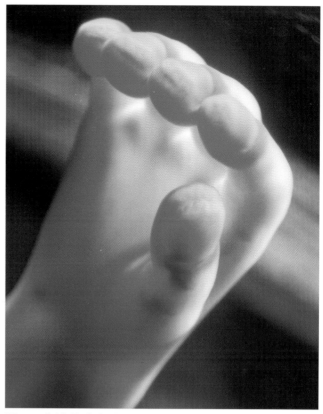

Figure 8.11 Early fetal hand: the fingers with nails

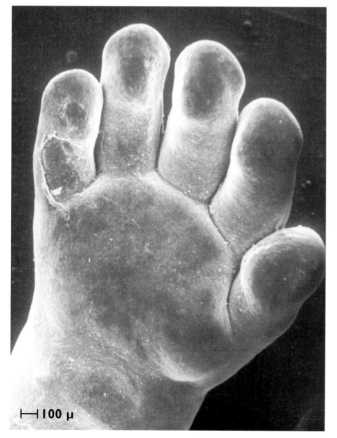

Figure 8.12 Hand with differentiated fingers of a late embryo, 54 days old (scanning electron microscopy)

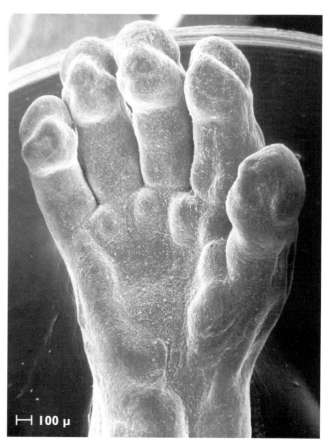

Figure 8.13 Hand with fingers exhibiting distinct volar pads: characteristic of embryos with fusing eyelids and of early fetuses, weeks 10–12 (scanning electron microscopy)

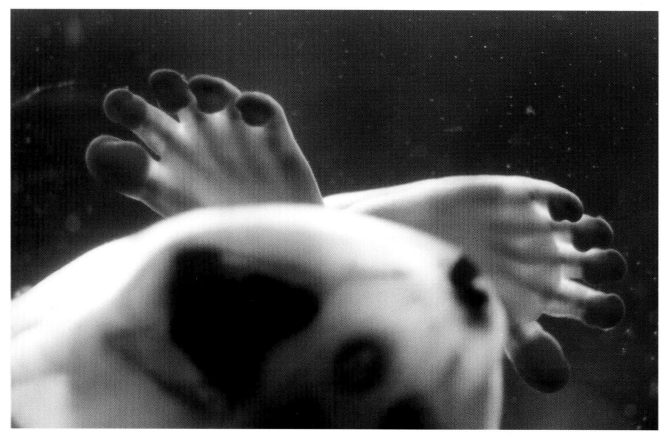

Figure 8.14 Toes with volar pads in an early fetus from the 11th gestational week

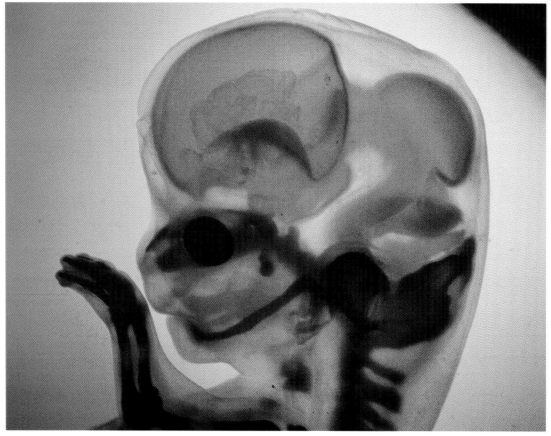

Figure 8.15 Chondrocranium (head skeleton) and brain in a 56-day-old embryo

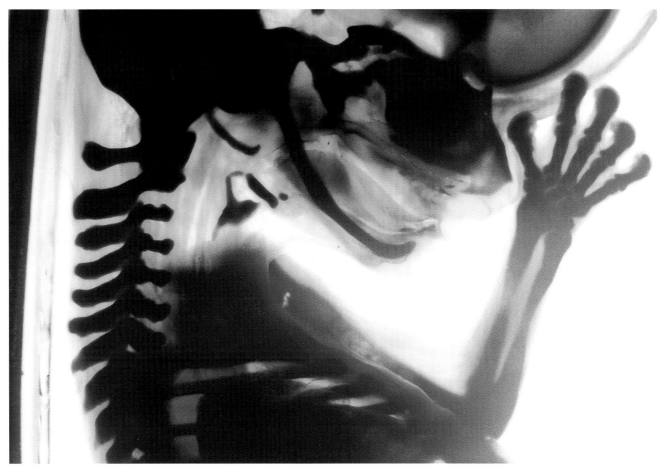

Figure 8.16 Cartilaginous skeleton in a fetus from the 16th gestational week

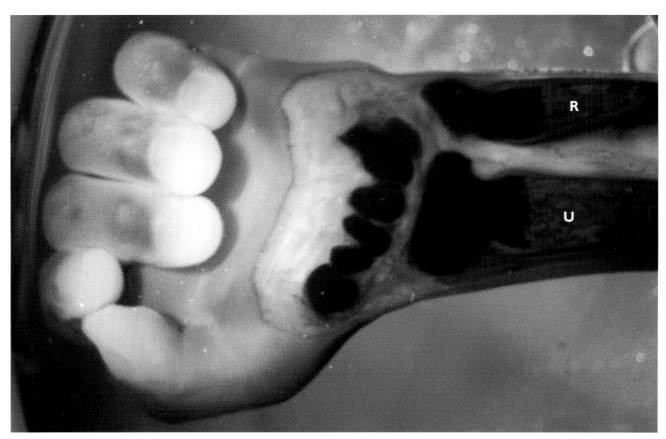

Figure 8.17 Dissected hand of a fetus from the 18th gestational week: the cartilaginous models of bones (blue) are replaced by bone tissue (red). Ossifiying distal portions of the antebrachium (ulna (U) and radius (R)) are evident

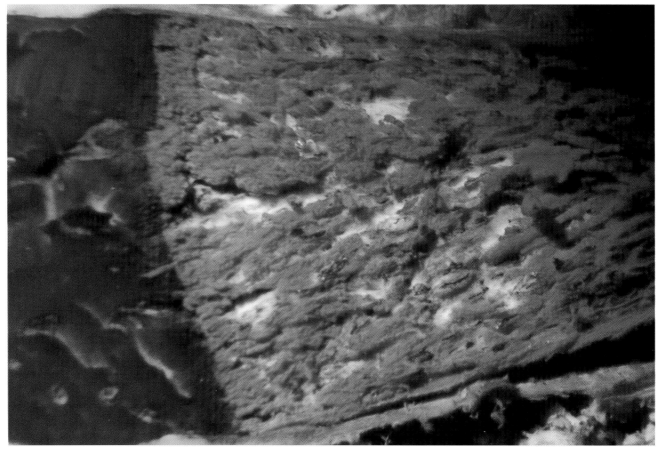

Figure 8.18 Advanced ossification of the fetal femur: cartilage appears blue, osseous alkaline phosphatase appears red

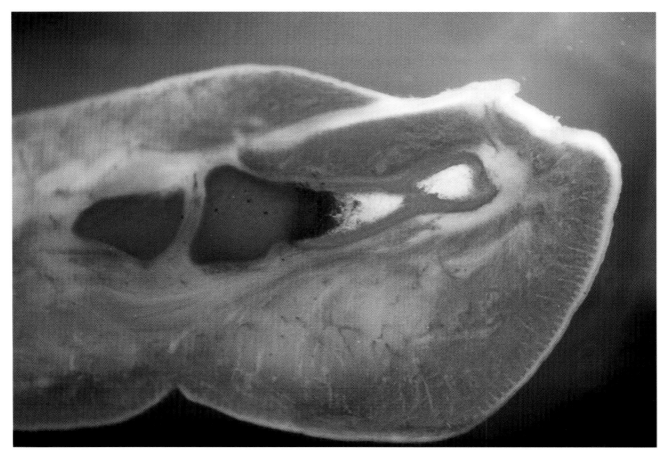

Figure 8.19 Anatomy of fetal finger at 20 weeks: the ossified portion of the terminal phalanx appears red, the cartilaginous portion appears blue. The nail plate is located dorsally on the terminal portion of the finger

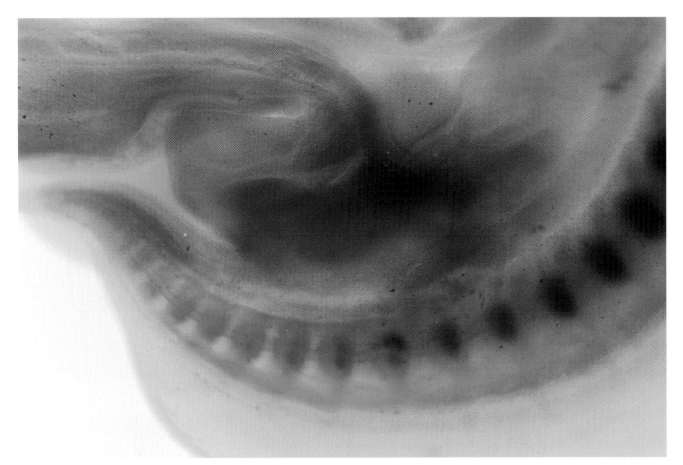

Figure 8.20 Terminal portion of the cartilaginous vertebral column in a 42-day-old (12 mm) embryo: vertebrae (dark blue) and intervertebral disks (light blue) are formed around the notochord

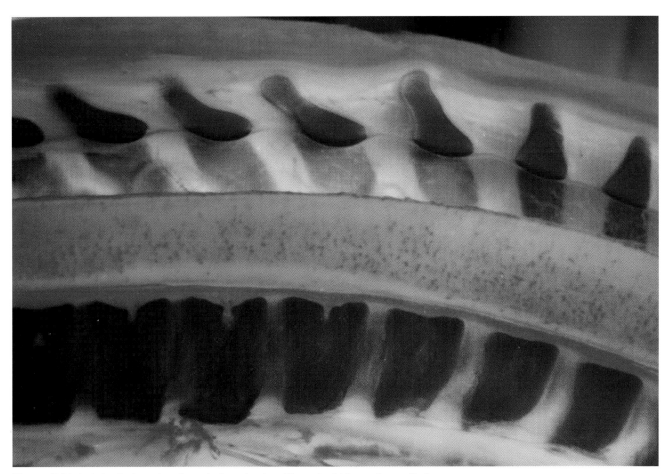

Figure 8.21 Longitudinal section through the spine in a 12-week-old fetus: the cartilaginous vertebrae appear blue, the medullary tube appears red

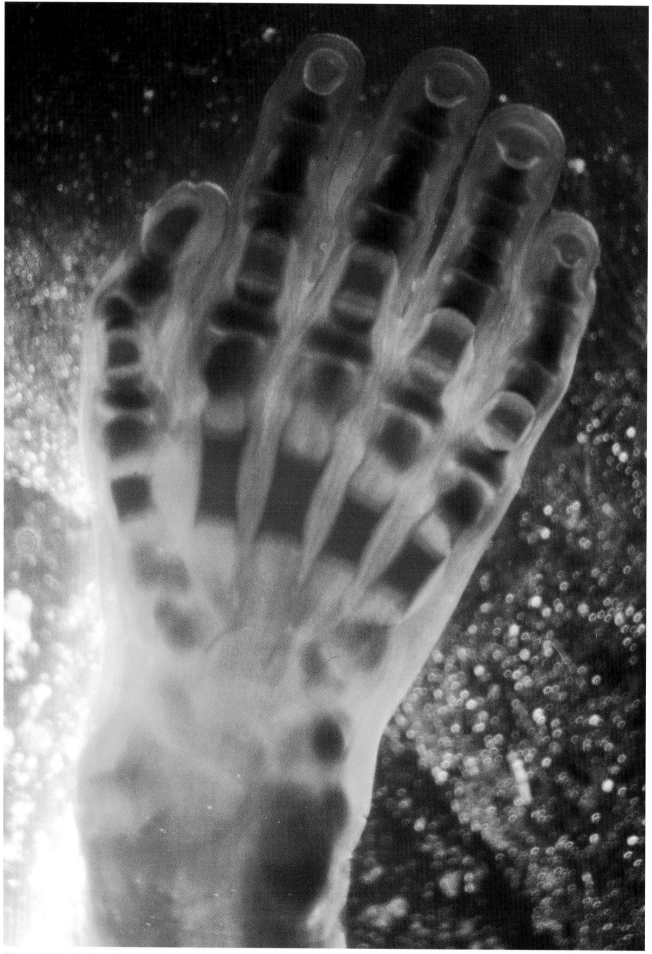

Figure 8.22 Ossifying fetal hand at the 20th gestational week: cartilages are blue. Distinct zones of ossification can be seen: each zone is encircled by a transparent halo. The bone trabeculae (red) are located within these zones

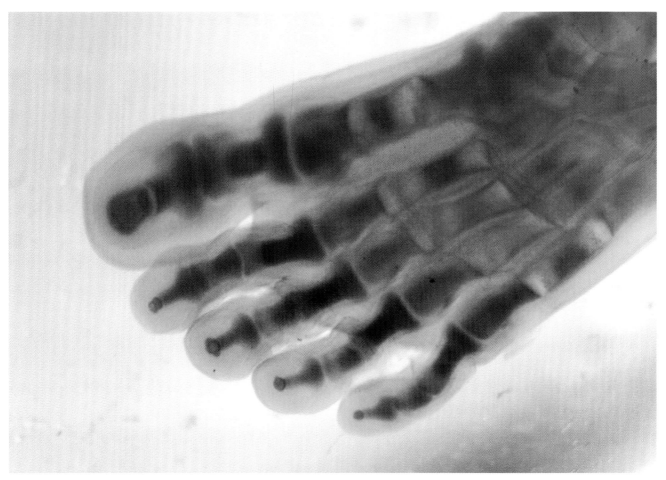

Figure 8.23 Ossifying foot of the same fetus as the hand shown in Figure 8.22

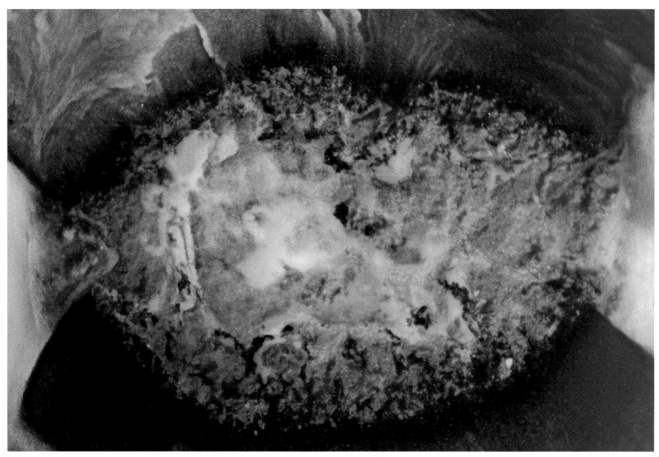

Figure 8.24 Ossification center within a cartilaginous vertebra: the osseous alkaline phosphatase is stained red

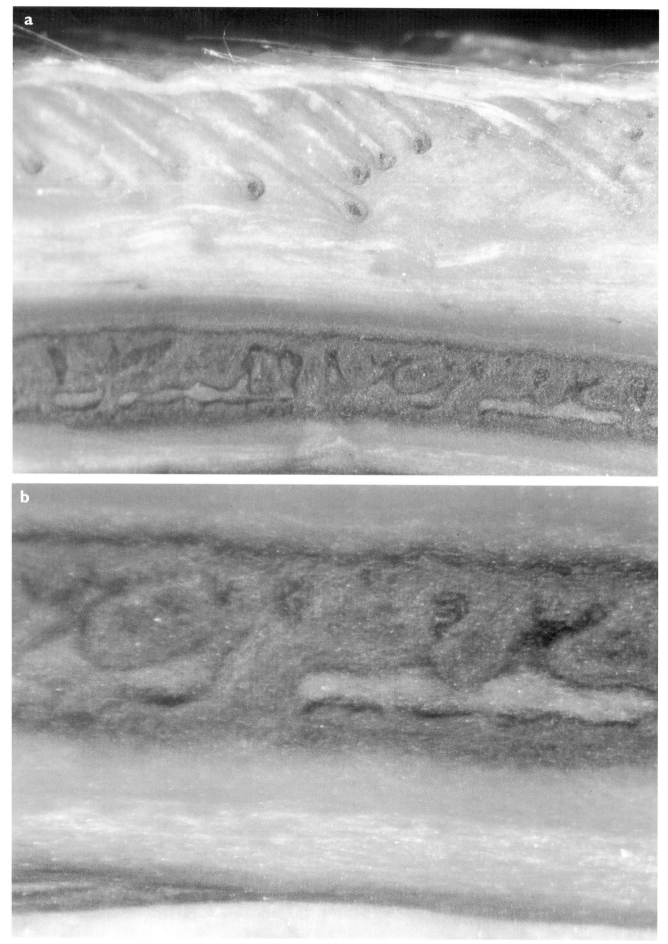

Figure 8.25 (a) Structure of a parietal bone (red) of a 20-week-old fetus: ossification of flat bones of the skull is desmogenic and occurs within connective tissue under the skin, without any preformed cartilage; (b) represents a detail from (a)

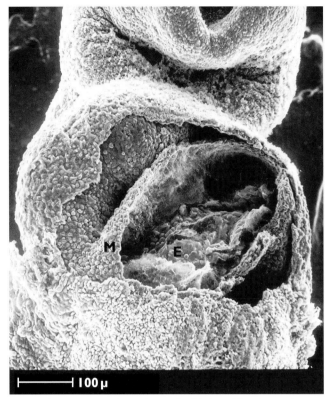

Figure 9.1 Dissected heart loop of a 24-day-old embryo: the loop consists of the myocardial mantle (M) with cardiac jelly, and the endothelial tube (E) (scanning electron microscopy)

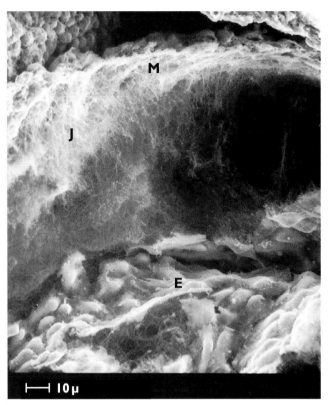

Figure 9.2 Myocardial mantle (M), cardiac jelly (J) and endothelial tube (E) of the heart tube (scanning electron microscopy)

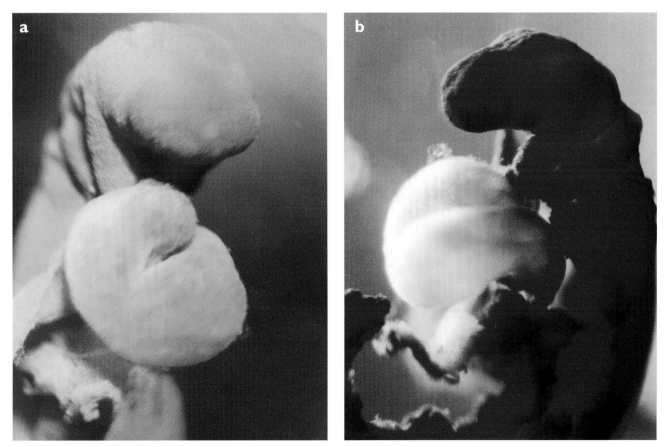

Figure 9.3 Heart loop of a 29–30-day-old (3.5 mm) embryo: (a) anterior view: the loop is left convex. The interface between the atrial and ventricular segments of the loop is delineated on the concave outline of the loop by the early interventricular sulcus; (b) heart loop viewed from the left side

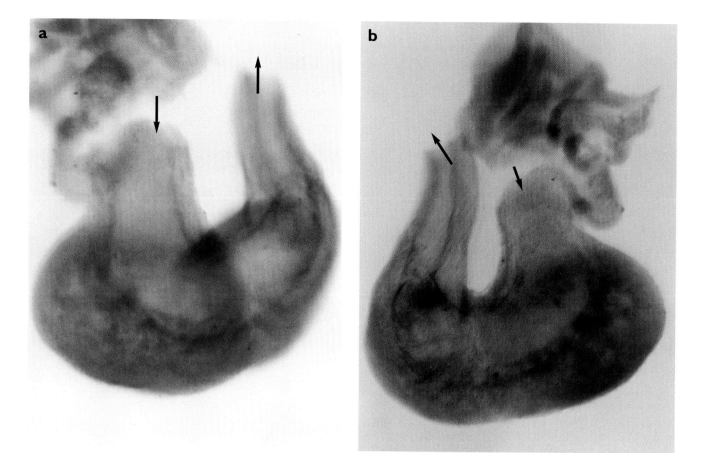

Figure 9.4 Dissected isolated heart loop from a 31–32-day-old (approximately 4 mm) embryo: the subendocardial layer appears blue because of the cardiac jelly. The thickened myoepicardial mantle (brown) on the convex side of the loop represents the myocardial basket. (a) Posterior view; (b) anterior view. The blood flow is marked with arrows

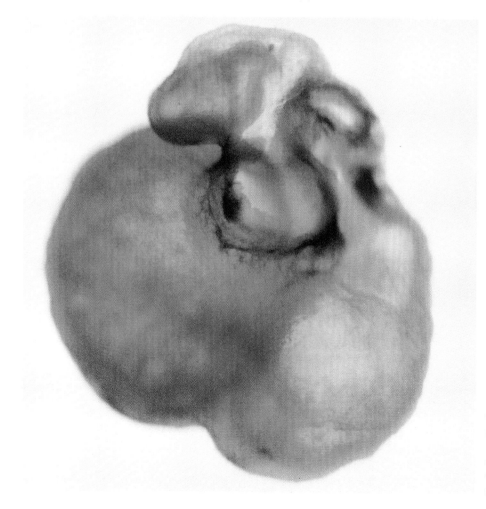

Figure 9.5 Segmentation of the heart in a 35-day-old (8 mm) embryo: view from the dorsal side. The right atrium and the venous sinus have been removed. Note the common atrioventricular opening, the left ventricle, the right ventricle and the aortopulmonary segment

a

b

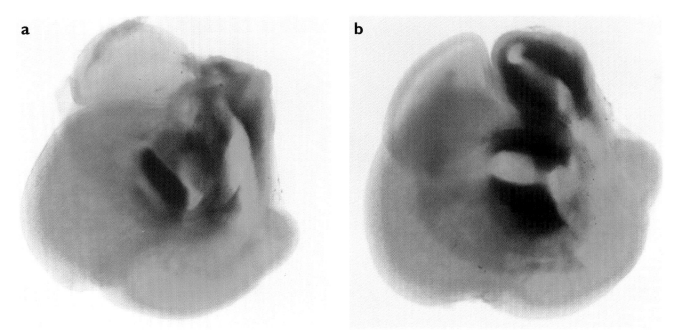

Figure 9.6 Septation of the heart in a 36-day-old (9 mm) embryo: the atrioventricular opening and the spiral folds of the aortopulmonary segment of the bulbus are evident. (a) Viewed from the dorsal side, the atrioventricular cushions precede formation of the valves; (b) the spiral folds separating the aortopulmonary segment

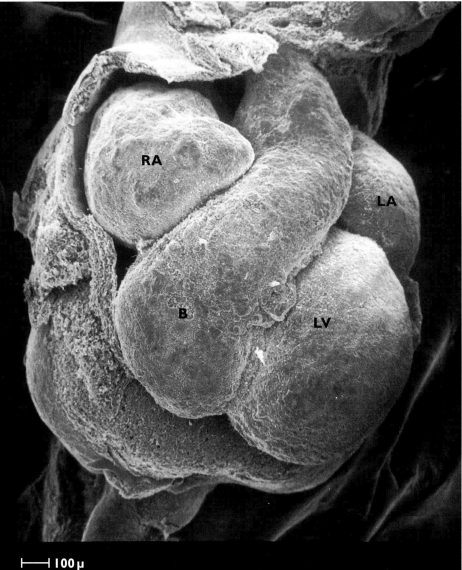

100 μ

Figure 9.7 Heart of a 37–38-day-old (8 mm) embryo, scanning electron microscopy (RA – right atrium; LA – left atrium; LV – left ventricle; B – bulbus)

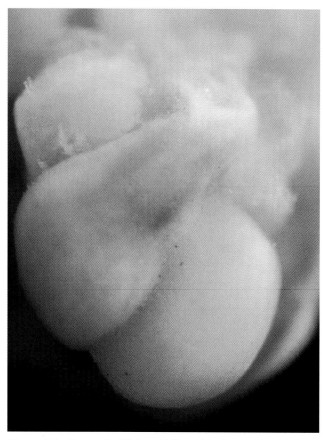

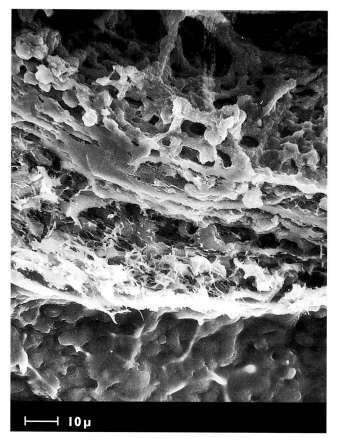

Figure 9.8 Heart of a 37-day-old (9 mm) embryo: anterior view visualizing the right and left atria, both ventricles and the aortopulmonary segment (blue). The red indistinct spots located between the left atrium and left ventricle and between both ventricles and the aortopulmonary segment are related to innervation

Figure 9.9 Embryonic heart wall: endomyocardium and epicardium (scanning electron microscopy)

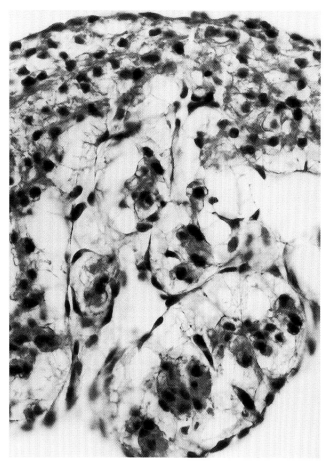

Figure 9.10 Histological section of embryonic heart ventricle: the epicardium, the myocardium (red) and the cardiac jelly (blue), which provides substratum for the endothelium, lining the cavity

a

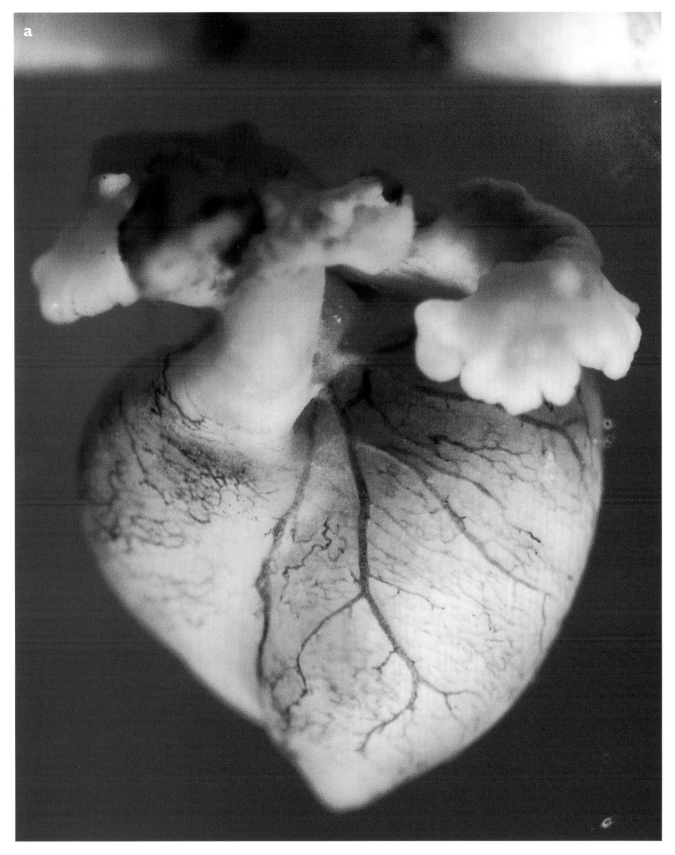

Figure 9.11 Heart of a 44-day-old (15 mm) embryo: anterior view. (a) Prominent auricles bulge
from both atria. Coronary vessels (black, arteries black-red), seen in the subepicardial region on
the surface of both ventricles, nourish the myocardium (scale marks millimeter intervals)

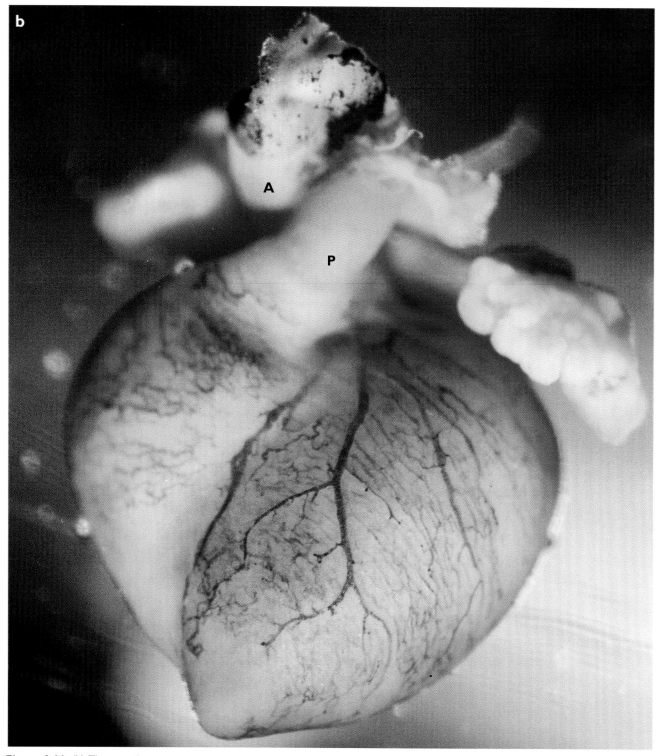

Figure 9.11 (b) The same heart showing positions of the pulmonary artery (P) and the aorta (A)

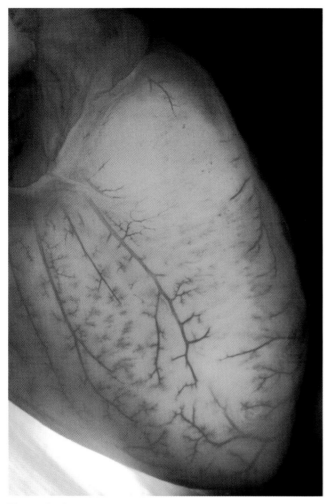

Figure 9.12 Heart of a 42–44-day-old (12 mm) embryo exhibiting angiogenesis: growing coronary arteries appear red

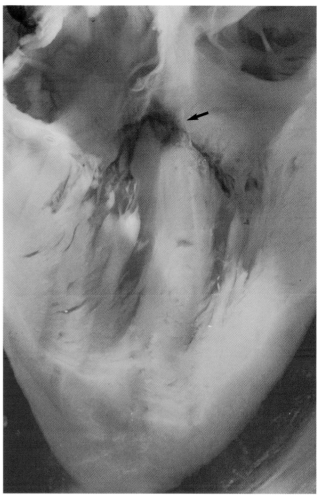

Figure 9.13 The four chambers of the fetal heart: between the right atrium and the right ventricle can be seen the tricuspid valve. The right and left atria are incompletely separated by membranous septum primum and muscular septum secundum. The fissure between the two septa is known as the foramen ovale. Between the left atrium and the left ventricle can be seen the mitral (bicuspid) valve. Both ventricles are separated by a thick muscular septum, except a small portion (blue) located between the right ventricle and left atrium, contributed by a membranous septum (arrow)

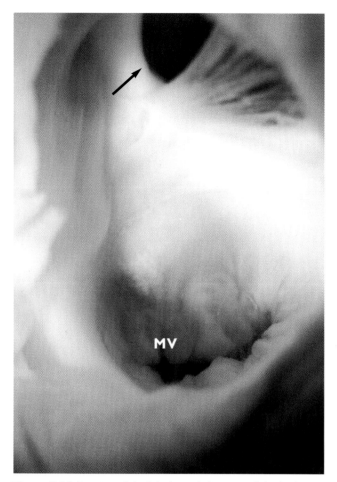

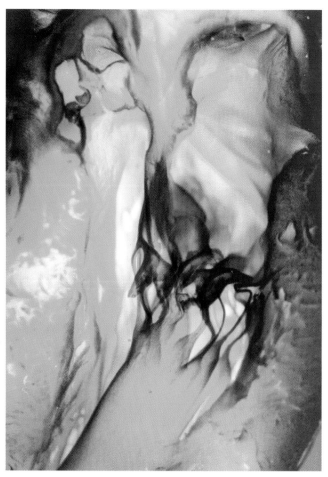

Figure 9.14 Interior of the left distended atrium of the fetal heart: the interatrial communication, the foramen ovale (arrow in the upper portion of the photograph) is delineated by the fleshy septum secundum (left) and by a membranous septum primum (right). The atrioventricular opening (entrance into the left ventricle) is closed by the mitral valve (MV) (in the lower portion of the photograph)

Figure 9.15 Interior of the left ventricle of the fetal heart: tendons of the papillary muscle are attached to the mitral valve. In the left upper corner can be seen the semilunar valves of the aorta; in the right upper corner can be seen the atrioventricular opening

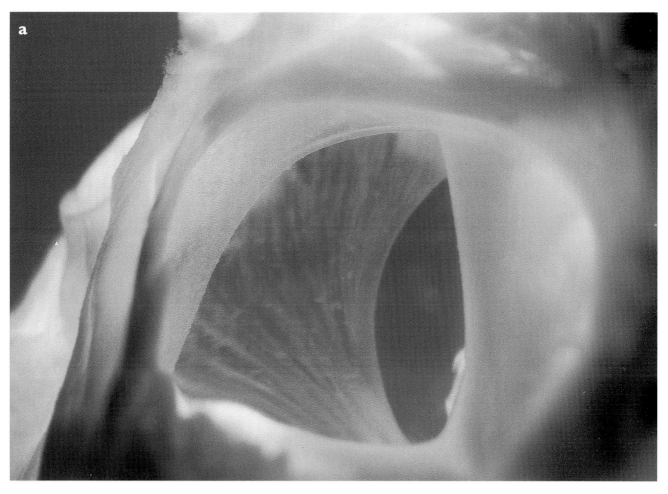

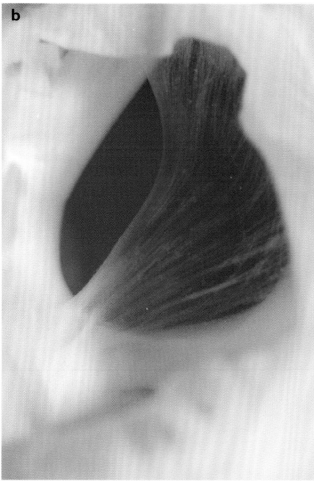

Figure 9.16 Interatrial foramen delineated by the thick septum secundum and a thin, membranous, septum primum: both atria are distended. (a) View from the right atrium; (b) view from the left atrium

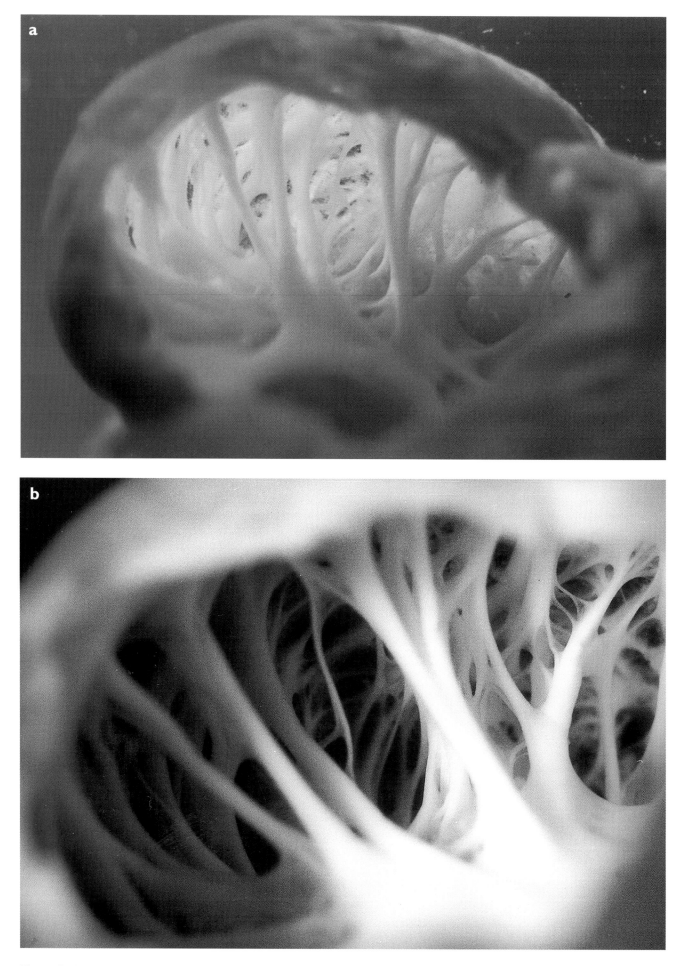

Figure 9.17 Architecture of pectinate muscles within the auricle of the left atrium of the
fetal heart: (a) translucent view; (b) pattern of pectinate muscles bridging the auricle

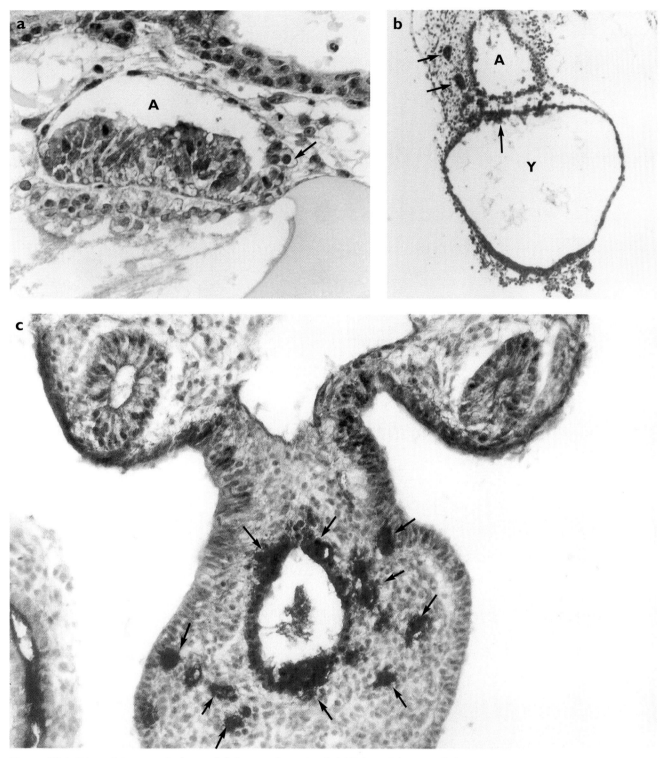

Figure 10.1 Primordial germ cells (arrows) (microscopic sections). (a) Primordial germ cells in a 13.5-day-old blastocyst: the cells are caudal to the ectoblast in the adjacent portion of the amniotic sac (A). The germ disk is bilaminar with a primary yolk sac. (b) Migrating primordial germ cells (red) in the early trilaminar embryo (days 16–17): primordial germ cells are present in the mesenchyme of the connecting stalk and invade the caudal portion of the ceiling of the yolk sac (Y). (c) In somite embryos with limb buds (32–35 days), primordial germ cells migrate from the endoderm of the gut into the mesenchyme of the mesentery and to the urogenital ridges. There are no sex differences related to the identification and migration of primordial germ cells

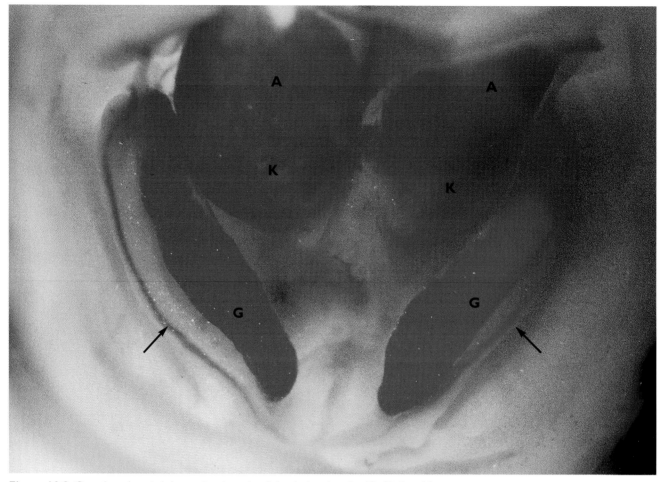

Figure 10.2 Gonads and genital ducts: view into the abdominal cavity of a 48–49-day-old (18 mm) embryo. The gonadal ridges (G) (embryonic ovaries, red) are elongated organs attached to the mesonephric ridges. Müllerian ducts (red lines, arrows) are located at the lateral margin of the mesonephric ridges. Large fetal adrenals (A) apposed to the kidneys (K) are present on both sides of the mesentery

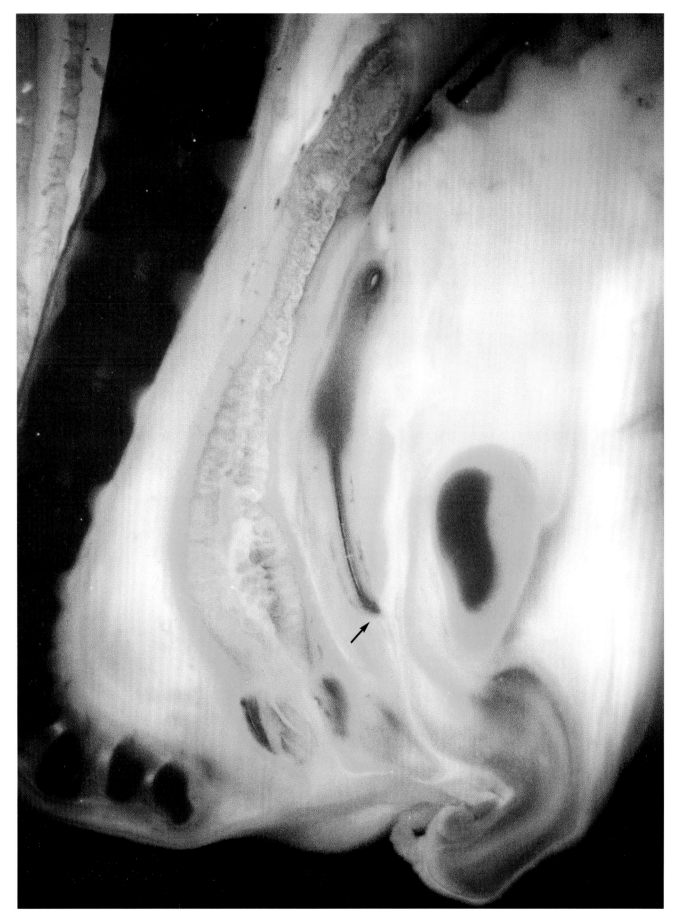

Figure 10.3 Midline sagittal dissection showing the anatomy of the female pelvis in the fetus
from the 12th gestational week: the position of the following organs is evident: descending colon,
rectum and anus. The uterovaginal canal (primordium of the uterus and vagina) is attached to the
urogenital sinus at the paramesonephric tubercle (arrow). The urinary bladder, symphysis of the
pelvic bones and the clitoris are visualized

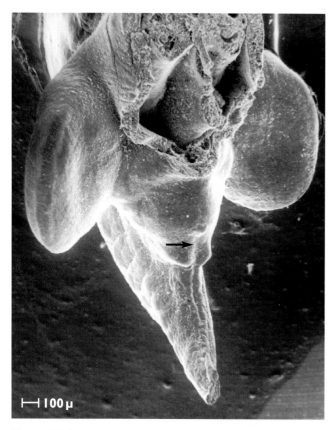

Figure 10.4 Hypogastric area with cloacal membrane (arrow) and anal hillocks of a 36-day-old embryo with limb buds (scanning electron microscopy)

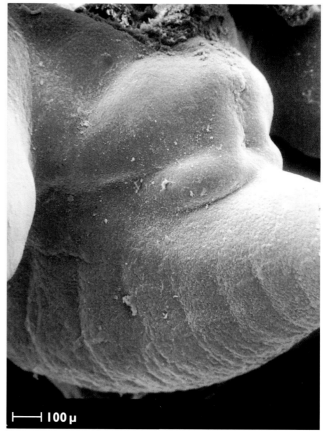

Figure 10.5 Genital tubercle in a 42-day-old embryo (scanning electron microscopy)

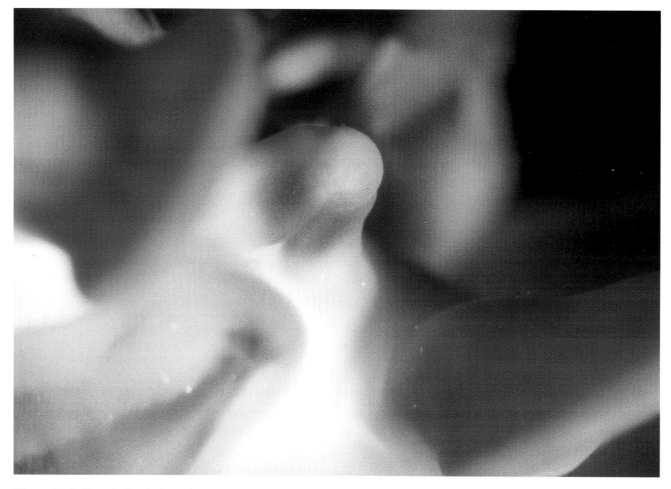

Figure 10.6 Genital tubercle located anterior to the tail in a 45-day-old embryo

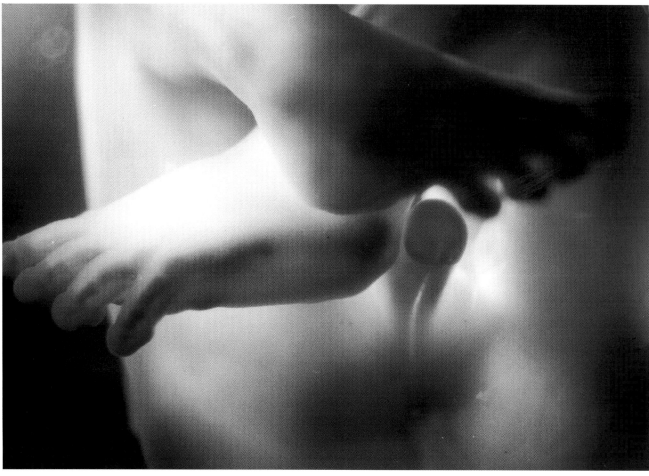

Figure 10.7 Phallus in a 56-day-old (28 mm) embryo

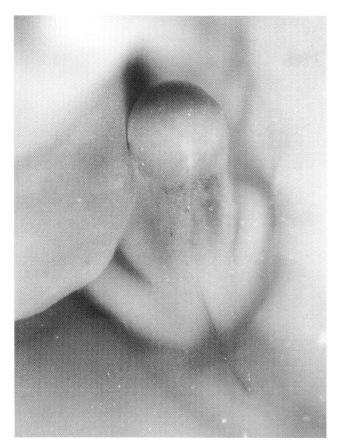

Figure 10.8 Early male transformation of external genitalia: the caudal ends of the labioscrotal folds become apposed at the midline. The anogenital distance increases

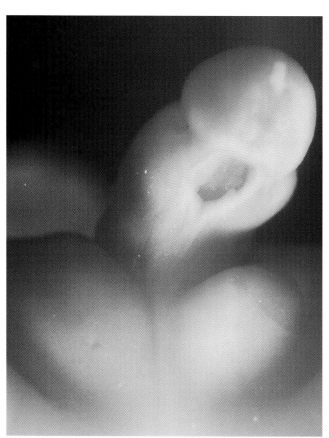

Figure 10.9 Closing of the male penile urethra by two streams of mesenchyme on each side: the medially located streams close the urethra, the lateral streams close the skin

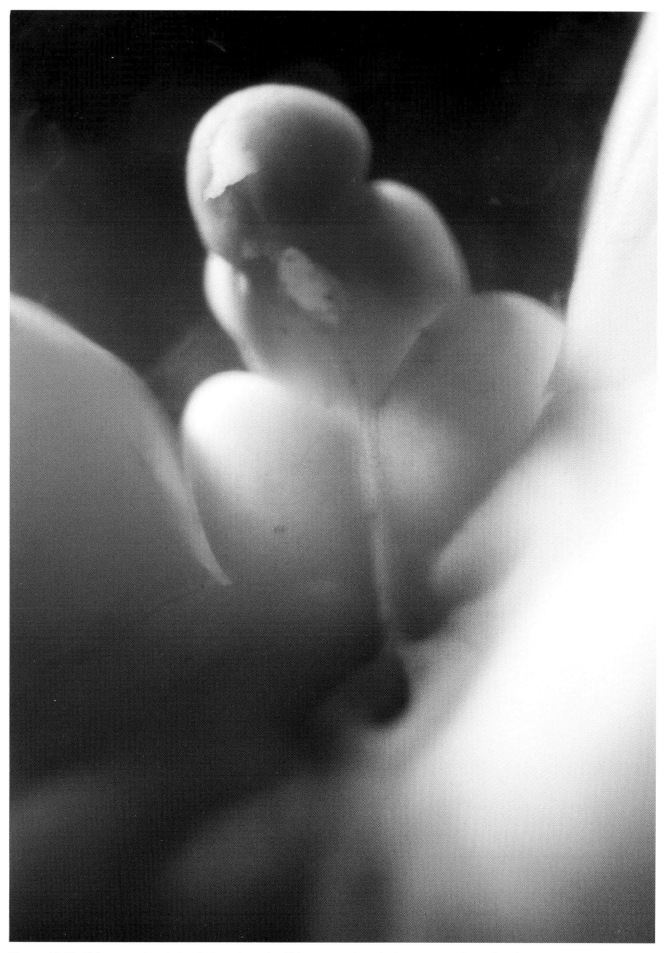

Figure 10.10 Male external genitalia of a fetus from the 13th gestational week: the scrotum is formed as the raphe connects adjacent portions of the labioscrotal folds. The penile urethra closes; the glans of the penis exhibits a midline epithelial plate with a distinct epithelial plug

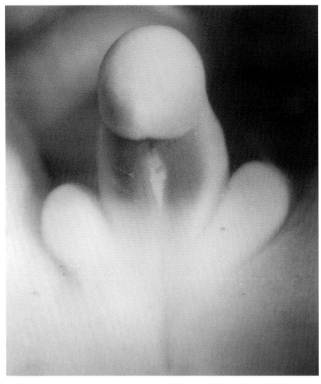

Figure 10.11 Early feminization of the phallus: the phallic urethra bends ventrally. No raphe is formed either between the labioscrotal folds or between the rims of the urethral groove

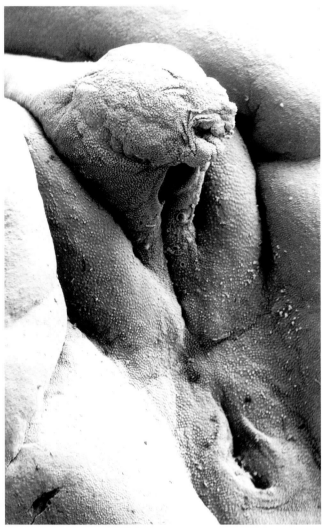

Figure 10.12 Normal female external genitalia at the 14th gestational week (scanning electron microscopy)

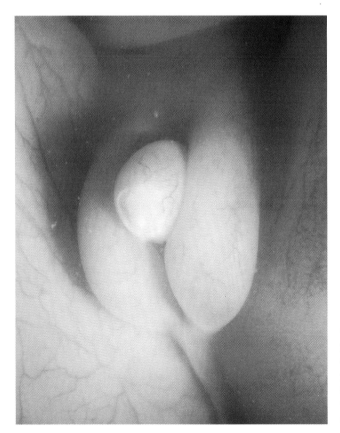

Figure 10.13 Malformed external genitalia of an 18-week-old female fetus: the mother was exposed to testosterone during gestational weeks 12 and 13. The labioscrotal folds and the clitoris are enlarged, but no raphe has formed. At 12 gestational weeks, the distance between the urethral opening and the dorsal commissure of the labioscrotal folds prevents formation of the scrotal and penile raphe, even in the presence of the male sex hormone in a testosterone-sensitive fetus

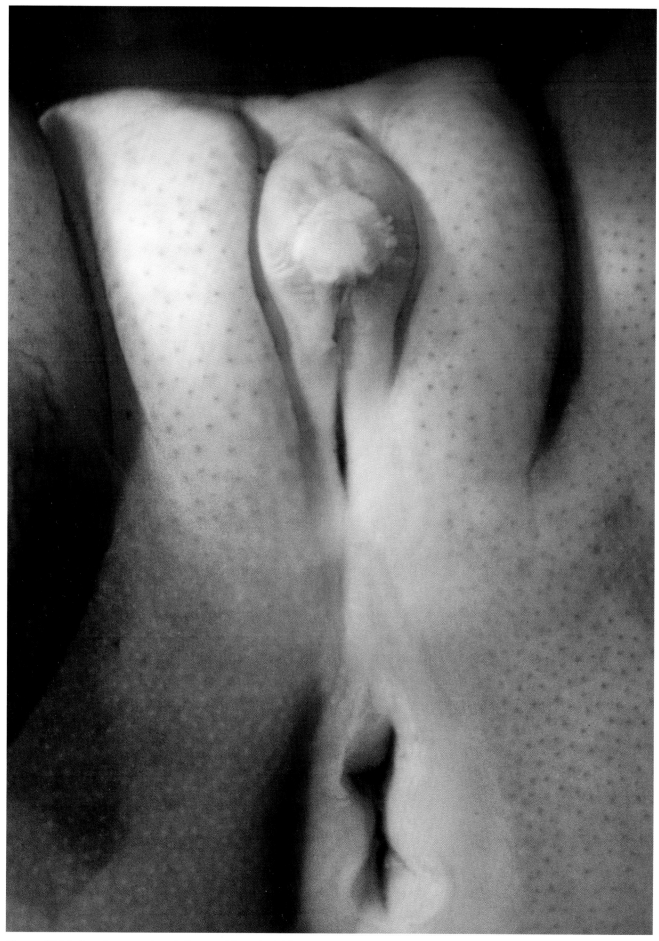

Figure 10.14 Female external genitalia in an 18-week-old fetus: the phallus changes into the clitoris. The rims of the urethral groove give rise to the labia minora; the labioscrotal folds transform into the labia majora. Red dots are developing hair follicles

INDEX

Page numbers in **bold** refer to figures.